HARDSTYLE ABS

Hit Hard. Lift Heavy. Look the Part.

By Pavel

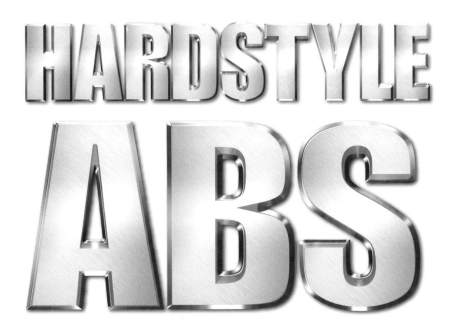

By Pavel

Published in the United States by:
Dragon Door Publications, Inc
5 East County Rd B, #3 • Little Canada, MN 55117
Tel: (651) 487-2180 • Fax: (651) 487-3954
Credit card orders: 1-800-899-5111
Email: support@dragondoor.com • Website: www.dragondoor.com

ISBN 10: 0-938045-50-4   ISBN 13: 978-0-938045-50-2

This edition first published in September, 2012

Printed in China

Book design, and cover by Derek Brigham
Website http//www.dbrigham.com • Tel/Fax: (763) 208-3069 • Email: bigd@dbrigham.com

DISCLAIMER
The author and publisher of this material are not responsible in any manner whatsoever for any injury that may occur through following the instructions contained in this material. The activities, physical and otherwise, described herein for informational purposes only, may be too strenuous or dangerous for some people and the reader(s) should consult a physician before engaging in them.

The author would like to thank the following individuals for their suggestions for this manuscript:

Dr. Mark Cheng
Bret Contreras
Jon Engum
Prof. Tom Fahey
Steve Freides
Brad Johnson
Brett Jones
Jeremy Layport
Prof. Stuart McGill
Gary Music
Jeff O'Connor
Mark Reifkind
m.c. schraefel
Chad Waterbury

WARNING

THIS BOOK IS NOT FOR YOU IF YOU HAVE ANY
OF THE FOLLOWING:

- HIGH BLOOD PRESSURE
- HEART CONDITION
- FLEXION INTOLERANT LOWER BACK

—TABLE OF CONTENTS—

Introduction:
The Mission

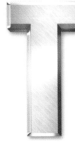his book has one goal—an extraordinarily strong and developed "six-pack"—and no other.

On these pages you will not find planks and other accoutrements of "functional training". Not because they are useless—far from it—but because they are unable to produce real "body armor". Don't blame a fork for being a poor knife.

Hardstyle Abs unapologetically applies to ab development the proven strength training methodologies of the world's best lifters, from the lighter weight classes. To be exact, to three exceptional exercises—reverse engineered from the body language of elite gymnasts.

Failing to train your abdominals for strength has been one of your downfalls. Getting distracted by what Mark Reifkind calls "random acts of variety" is another. Instead of spreading yourself thin over dozens of ineffective moves you shall laser focus on three killer drills.

If you follow the instructions to the letter, I guarantee results. Noticeable within weeks. Extraordinary within months.

Hit hard. Lift heavy. Look the part.

HARDSTYLE
ABS

- **Three Killer Moves**

- **Pure Strength Methodology**

- **Old Time Strongman Mindset**

- **Ancient Martial Arts Breathing Technique**

- **Reverse-Engineered Body Language of an Elite Gymnast**

Rigor mortis, or why high reps have failed you

You tried high reps. You went for the "burn". It did not work. Why do you insist on doing the same thing and expect a different outcome?

The "burn" you feel from high reps is from lactate buildup and does absolutely nothing for toning up your muscles. I remember picking up a copy of *The Guinness Book of World Records* and seeing a picture of the gent who held the record for the number of consecutive sit-ups—many, many thousands. This martyr must have "felt the burn" more than anyone else on this planet, yet he did not even have a six-pack to show for it, in spite of his low level of body fat.

To know why high reps have failed this Comrade and many others, one must understand what makes abs hard and strong. It is a **combination of increased resting tension or tonus and "real" muscle growth.**

Muscle tone is simply residual tension in a relaxed muscle. And tension is the means by which a muscle generates force. The more tiny strands of contractile proteins hook on to each other, the more tension and force the muscle produces, the more tone it exhibits. Contrary to popular belief, a resting muscle is not totally relaxed—your body would have collapsed into a bag of bones if it were—but partially tensed, preloaded to spring into action.

The English words "tone" and "tune" were derived from the same Old French word: *ton*. It is no surprise that muscle tone has been poetically likened to the tautness of a guitar string. Think of "toned" muscles as "tuned for action".

Of course, one must differentiate between tight muscles and toned muscles. The former are short and stiff, the latter long and vibrant, ready to go off like a drawn bow. Stand up and imagine that you are about to get punched in the stomach. Brace your abs without hunching over. This is what good muscle tone feels like.

Muscles get short because they don't get much of an opportunity to be long. One scenario is inactivity and bad posture. When a person spends a lot of time sitting, his abs shorten. Because he is lazy, they also weaken. As they get weaker, they get tighter.

In another scenario, the person does strength train but only through a short range of motion: consider the permanently bent arms of a bodybuilder.

The third scenario is akin to rigor mortis. Your muscle fibers are like mousetraps—they go off by themselves, but need energy to be reset to contract again. A dead body is out of ATP, the energy compound that relaxes the muscles. Thus the muscles of a "stiff" are permanently contracted. A typical high rep ab workout exhausts ATP in the muscles and they lock up like those of a dead man. This is spasm, not tone, and it is produced by popular abdominal routines. Such "zombie tone" does not last—you have to "kill" the muscles day in and day out with mind numbing reps.[1]

Like a mousetrap that has already fired but cannot be reset, a short, tight muscle is worthless in sports.

A muscle with a healthy muscle tone will also have a substantial number of fibers that are active at all times—but at a greater length. The mousetrap is loaded.

To acquire such tonus one must do three things.

First, **train the muscles with high tension.** It should be apparent that one cannot maintain high levels of tension for a long period of time. Over decades of experience, strength coaches have determined that five reps are about all one can do and fewer are just fine.

Second, **prevent the muscle from shortening:**

    a) **Stretching after strength training;**
    b) **Doing at least some strength exercises through a long range of motion;**
    c) **Training the antagonists (the back extensors in the abs' case)**

Healthy muscle tone is the first prerequisite for rock hard abs; "real" muscle growth is the other.

There are two types of muscular hypertrophy: *sarcoplasmic* and *myofibrillar*. The former increases the number of capillaries and blows the muscle up with glycogen and other energy compounds needed to endure the demands of high reps. And one molecule of glycogen binds three molecules of water. Now you know what bodybuilders' bloated bi's are made of. The latter, spurred by heavy resistance, increases the size of the fibers' contractile apparatus or *myofibrils*—the "real" muscle of a lifter or gymnast.

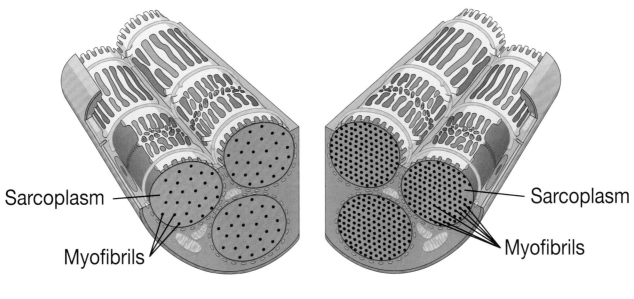

Sarcoplasm

Myofibrils

Sarcoplasm

Myofibrils

Bloated muscle built through pumping up

Real muscle built through heavy lifting

"Which type of hypertrophy is going to develop depends on the nature of training," explains Prof. Evgeniy Ilyin. "Prolonged dynamic efforts with a small load lead to the first type of hypertrophy; large muscle tensions in isometric regime—to the hypertrophy of the second type."

What is fascinating about myofibrillar hypertrophy from the standpoint of looking good is, (I quote the Russian professor),"The muscle's cross section may change insignificantly, as what mostly changes is the density of packing of the myofibrils in the muscle fiber." In other words, heavy weights make muscles dense and hard but not really big. Doesn't this sound like the abs you are after?

Some will argue: "Why would I train the abs with low reps? These are slow twitch muscles!"

First, this may or may not be true as the research is inconsistent.[3] But we do know that there are large individual differences in the percentage of slow Type I fibers in the rectus abdominis or RA: 32-76%.[4]

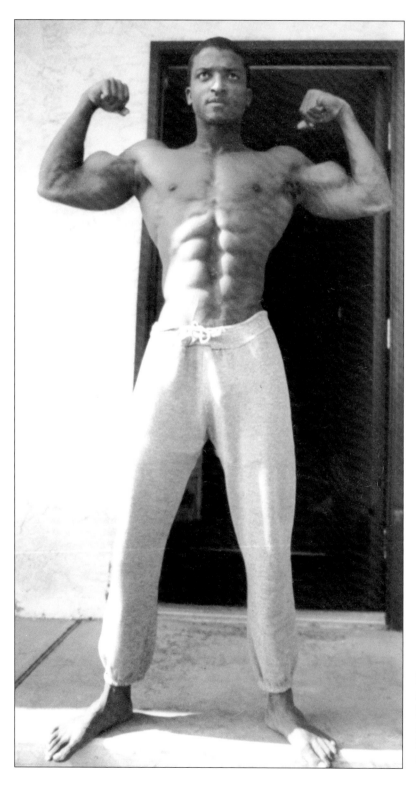

Second, your abbies' fiber composition is irrelevant. If your goals are strength and muscle definition you should go after your fast twitchers, whatever their percentage may be. Here is a fascinating gold nugget of research that has somehow escaped the eyes of bodybuilders for over four decades: faster muscle fibers congregate near the surface of the muscle and slower ones hide deep inside![5] Which could explain why lean strength athletes—powerlifters, weightlifters, gymnasts, etc.—display remarkably dense muscles and "high reppers" tend to stay soft.

Powerlifting champion Ausby Alexander proves the point that heavy lifting produces exceptional abs. Of course, they will show only if one stays lean as this Marine vet.
Photo courtesy Powerlifting USA

Bulgarian gymnastics coach Ivan Ivanov likes to say that low rep, heavy training "shrinks" muscles into one piece, while bodybuilding style pump-up "blows them up". It is instructive that Eugene Sandow, an iron legend equally famous for his strength and his physique, advised limiting the reps in abdominal exercises to three! Not surprisingly, he picked hard exercises like the straight arm, straight leg sit-up with dumbbells held overhead in straight arms.

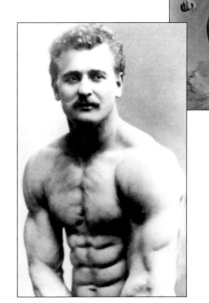

Third, I presume you want your abs to play the part, not just look the part. Muscle size is only half of the strength equation. The other half is the nervous system's ability to recruit the muscles and it can only be effectively developed with very brief efforts produced in a fresh state.[6]

Acquiring a killer six-pack becomes ridiculously simple and easy once you understand that you need to **train your midsection for strength and not endurance**. We have time tested simple and effective methodologies to do just that.

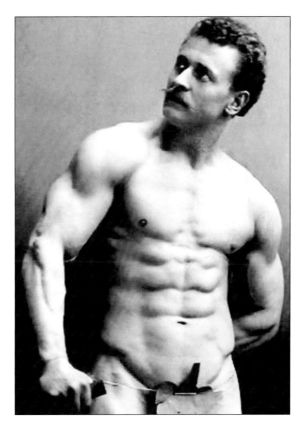

Eugene Sandow, an iron legend equally famous for his strength and his physique.

Getting that Six-Pack to Show

A Russian gave his friend a critical look: "Boy, you sure are getting fat, Comrade!"

The big Comrade finished chewing a piece of salted pork lard and responded pensively: "I aim for perfection! And what is the most perfect shape in the universe?" He paused for effect. "…The sphere!"

If this is not your idea of perfect shape, you had better lose the spare tire before taking on the *Hardstyle Abs* plan. Hardstyle breathing is not a good idea for heavy folks as they run a tendency towards high blood pressure and as for the Hardstyle sit-ups, your belly will quite literally get in the way. I am not even going to mention the hanging leg raise.

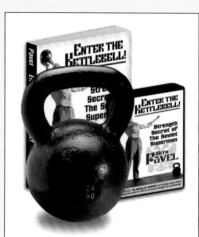

**Men's 35lb Russian Kettlebell
Quick-Start Kit with DVD
www.dragondoor.com/kkb009/**

How to lose fat?—The keys are kettlebell swings and smarter eating. My book and DVD *Enter the Kettlebell!* will teach you the former. Someone else will teach you the latter.

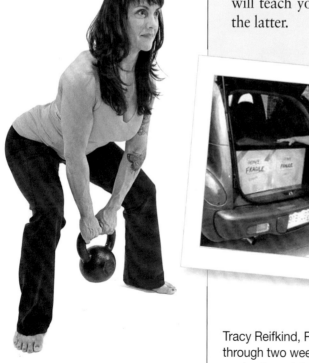

Tracy Reifkind, RKC lost 115 pounds through two weekly kettlebell swing workouts and better eating.
Before photo courtesy Tracy Reifkind

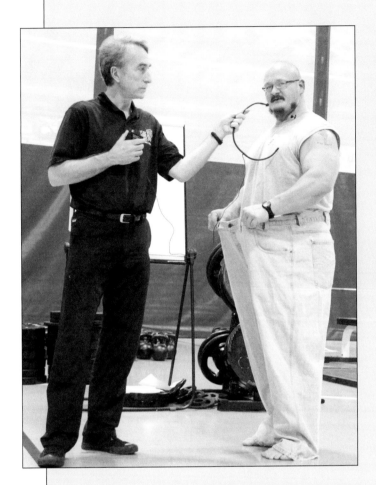

If you are already fairly lean, your upper abs are showing but the lower ones are not, the answer is losing even more fat. *Aponeuroses*, fibrous sheets performing the role of tendons for the obliques and transversus abdominis, pass over the six-pack beneath your belly button. So building and toning will not do much good there.

And as long as we are on the topic of the "upper" and "lower" abs, the top and the bottom of your rectus abdominis are indeed innervated sep-

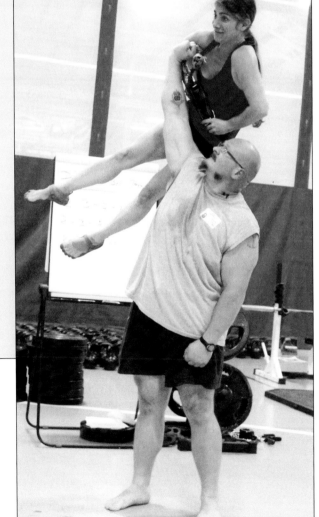

arately. However, scientists cannot come to an agreement whether this means anything to your midsection training. Some believe that only in low intensity contractions may the lower or the upper abs be isolated. Others are convinced that well coordinated subjects can pull it off.[7] Regardless, load the abs enough, and the whole length of your six-pack will light up like a Christmas tree.

Professional strongman Bud Jeffries, RKC also dropped 115 pounds, most of it fat, through kettlebell swing specialization. "I've maintained all, or almost all of my strength... Interestingly I actually gained strength in several areas... massively gained grip strength... gained a lot of back strength."

FOOTNOTES

1   "*Rigor mortis* is caused by lack of ATP, which is needed to pump calcium back into the sarcoplasmic reticulum. Calcium triggers muscle contractions and must be withdrawn to allow the muscle to relax." (Fahey, 2010)

2   Ilyin (2003)

3   Häggmark & Thorstensson (1979) reported that the RA is 55% slow twitch and Colling (1997) had the opposite results: 54% fast twitch.

4   Johnson et al. (1973), Colling-Saltin (1979)

5   Clamann (1970)

6   "An important maxim of muscle physiology is that a fiber is trained in direct proportion to its recruitment." (Fahey, 2010)

7   Bret Contreras comments: "My problem with the other researchers is that they weren't measuring the most effective movements to target the upper versus the lower abs. My experiments show that you can definitely target one over the other. I know McGill showed that belly dancers could completely isolate one over the other, so there is probably a neural aspect that can be learned over time. At any rate, I palpate the upper and lower abs of people doing RKC planks and you will definitely feel the low abs being rock hard with the upper not as hard, which is consistent with their posterior pelvic tilting role… research down the road might provide more definitive conclusions…"

Hardstyle Breathing:
how to shrink-wrap your waist with an ancient martial arts technique

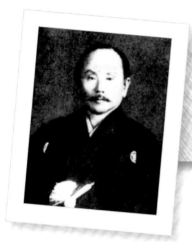

> TO SEARCH FOR THE OLD IS TO UNDERSTAND THE NEW.
> —GICHIN FUNAKOSHI

The first thing you are going to learn is how to breathe in a manner that compresses your viscera hard enough to make a diamond—Hardstyle breathe. Exercises of this type supposedly date 1,500 years back to Bodhidharma, semi-mythical progenitor of Asian martial arts. More importantly, they have been endorsed by top Russian scientists.[8]

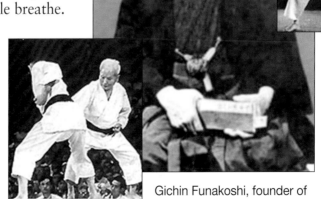

Gichin Funakoshi, founder of modern karate-do.

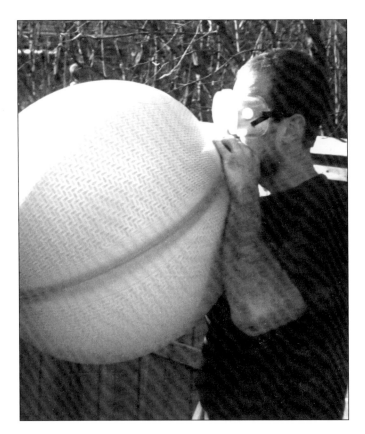

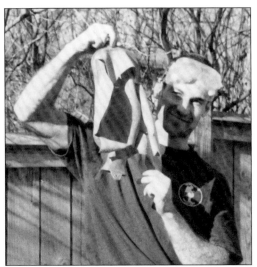

Testing the effectiveness of Hardstyle breathing. Don't try it at home. According to Don Ross, if you goof up and let the air pressure—up to 600 pounds according to the late Mr. America and performing strongman—back up into your lungs you could die from lung barotrauma. It reminds me of AVM-1, an old Soviet scuba rig… but I have digressed.

There are at least four reasons to Hardstyle breathe:

1. **For strength**
2. **For stronger activation of all midsection muscles**
3. **For back health**
4. **For a tighter waist**

First, for strength.

You will rarely if ever come across this reflex in Western literature: the *pneumo-muscular reflex*.[9] It can be compared to the amplifier of your stereo, where your brain is the record player and your muscles are the speakers. Special *baroreceptors* in your abdominal and thoracic cavities register the internal pressure and adjust your muscular tension like the volume control knob. The higher is this pressure, the greater your strength—and vice versa.

Martial artists have possessed the knowledge of this powerful reflex for centuries. A blood curdling "K-i-a-i!" does more than intimidate the opponent and raise the fighter's spirit. A sudden compression of the air by a powerful contraction of torso muscles peaks the intra-abdominal pressure (IAP) at the moment of the impact. This dramatically increases the power.

Second, for a stronger activation of all midsection muscles. The pneumo-muscular reflex alone will make your abs and obliques fire harder when you have squeezed your viscera with Hardstyle breathing. Another "muscle software app", *irradiation*, will make them tense even harder. When a muscle contracts intensely, its excitation spills over to its neighbors and gets them all worked up as well. "In union there is strength." So the fact that the muscles responsible for building up the IAP like the transversus and the internal obliques are working hard will make the abs, the external obliques, etc. work harder too.

Third, for back health.

The contraction of many muscles of the midsection stimulated by Hardstyle breathing strengthens these muscles and builds a strong brace for your back. And the fact that you are learning how to maximize the intra-abdominal pressure adds another protective mechanism, pneumatic-hydraulic. Just imagine how much more impervious your spine would be if instead of wiggly inner organs you had a blown up tire in your abdomen! No need to imagine any more.[10]

Fourth, for a tighter waist.

The resistance created by Hardstyle breathing not only trains the superficial muscles of the abdominal wall but also the "warriors of the invisible front" like the transversus abdominis and the internal obliques.

You have heard a lot about the role of the TVA in back health and a tight looking waist. While this muscle does play a role in both, the common cues for activating it, to "suck your stomach in" or "pull the belly button towards the spine, are dangerous and ineffective.

Try this experiment. Stand up. Blow out all of your air, then, without taking any in, force your ribcage open. Your stomach has miraculously pulled in. What happened?—Opening the chest without inhaling makes the little air left in your lungs take up more space. That means low gas pressure. Nature abhors vacuum or anything close to it, so if air is unavailable, something else will rush in to fill the space. Your gut will do just that. The belly button is in. Without any help from the TVA.

Since high intra-abdominal pressure is essential for spine stability under load, "hollowing" is obviously a losing strategy for your squats and deadlifts. From the purely architectural point of view it does not make any sense either: a concave wall will collapse long before a straight one. I know lifters who fell for the hollowing fad in the nineties and they had nothing but injuries to show for it. Don't repeat their mistakes.

Even if lifting heavy things is not on your menu and looking good is all that matters—you big sissy!—you still want to up your IAP in your ab training because this happens to be one of the key functions of the TVA. Like a boa, it constricts your gut's contents.

But enough theory; let us get down to business.

Stand up with your knees slightly bent. Poke your fingers into your abs and obliques doing your best not to shrug your shoulders. Palpating your muscles will allow you to gauge their tension and thus tense them even more.

Take a diaphragmatic inhalation of approximately ½ to ¾ of the max volume. Pull air "...not [into] the upper stomach," stressed the late karate great Mas Oyama, "...force it into the groin. Force the air down, down... [and] force your feet... right through the ground."

If you have forgotten how to belly breathe as all kids do, practice the "crocodile breath" from the arsenal of Gray Cook, RKC and Brett Jones, Master RKC. The latter explains:

> *Begin lying face down with your forehead on your hands, both palms down, one covering the other. Make sure the chest and arms are relaxed and you are as "flat" as you can get; your neck should be neutral and comfortable.*

> *Breathe in through the nose and feel the air move down past the chest into the "stomach". When this happens, you will feel the abdomen push out against the ground. This should happen naturally without you forcing your stomach out.*

> *Exhale fully before beginning the next breath cycle.*

> *The key points:*
> * *Avoid breathing into the chest first and raising the shoulders.*
> * *Inhale and exhale through the nose at a natural pace taking 80% or larger inhalations and long exhalations.*
> * *You may exhale through the mouth.*
> * *Don't rush; there is a natural pause between the inhalation and exhalation cycles.*
> * *The floor will provide automatic proprioceptive feedback as the abdomen pushes out against it. It should also guide you to breathe into the obliques and into the back.*
> * *Perform 20-30 breaths in the beginning of a training session but shoot for 3-5 minutes of breath work at some later point.*

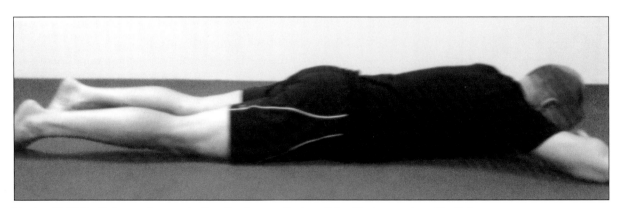

Master RKC Brett Jones demonstrating the "crocodile breath". *Photo courtesy Brett Jones*

Pull up your sphincters as if you are trying to restrain yourself from making both kinds of nature's calls. This maneuver, practiced for millennia in many martial arts, serves several purposes. To understand them you need to know a smidgen of anatomy.

Think of the area from your sternum down to the bottom of your pelvis as a box. The rectus abdominis (RA) or the "six-pack" is the front of the box, various back muscles are the back, the obliques are the sides. The top of the box is the diaphragm, a muscle that works like the plunger of a syringe. When it contracts and pushes down, it creates a lower pressure in the lungs, and you take an abdominal inhalation. The diaphragm also bears down to up your

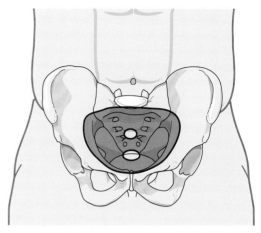

The Pelvic Floor

intra-abdominal pressure when you are lifting heavy weights. The bottom of the "box" is the pelvic diaphragm, which prevents the works from falling out and buys you time when you are looking for a bathroom.

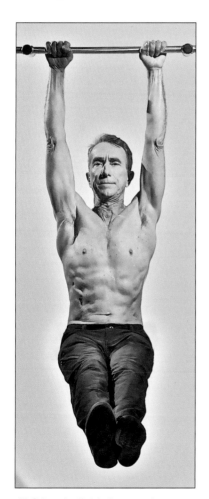

JDC has built his impressive abs with dynamic tension and Hardstyle breathing practices from Iron Shirt Qigong.

In our strength training practice we pull up the pelvic diaphragm and employ the "sphincter lock" for the duration of the strain. First, for health reasons. Although the pelvic floor muscles go live reflexively in response to an increased intra-abdominal pressure[11], a little extra insurance will not hurt. The late karate master Gogen Yamaguchi reportedly got some heavy-duty hemorrhoids for failing to employ the sphincter lock during his dynamic tension kata practice. The powerlifting community has its own share of horror stories. In addition to preventing the obvious, strengthening the pelvic floor (PF) muscles has some other health benefits that are outside of the scope of this book.

My friend and publisher John Du Cane, who has spent decades studying Chinese martial arts, offers useful pelvic floor training recommendations:

Many Qigong and Tai Chi masters recommend holding the perineum (area between anus and genitals) up the whole time you are practicing. Many recommend that you pull up the perineum throughout the day. If you get in the habit of gently pulling it up area as often and as much as you can, you will gradually become much more accomplished at isolating this key area and technique, for strength and energy preservation/generation. When you are then pulling up the perineum area in a more concentrated manner for particularly intense exercises like the squat or Iron Shirt Qigong, you will have developed a better ability to maintain the lock.

Second, because the pelvic diaphragm is an extra "compressor" which allows us to get the IAP even higher. And third, to amplify the tension of the abdominals reflexively. A contraction of the PF muscles automatically "lights up" the abs, obliques, and TVA.[12] Researchers poetically commented that "...contractions of the pelvic floor cast their shadow upon the abdominal muscles."[13]

So you have taken a 50-75% abdominal inhalation and pulled up your sphincters. Now press your tongue behind your teeth and hiss, trying to contract the abdomen as intensely as possible. It is important to press hard with your tongue in order to leave only a very small opening for the escaping air. Think of your mouth as the nozzle of an air hose. When it is relaxed, air flows out freely and builds up no pressure. But when you press your tongue against your teeth, as if to make the sound "TSSSSSSS!!!"(try pronouncing my last name), it is as if you have plugged the end of the hose with your thumb. Suddenly very little gas can escape and the pressure inside the tube goes way up. There are many types of pressurized or Hardstyle breathing. In the author's experience hissing is superior for forging a killer six-pack.[14]

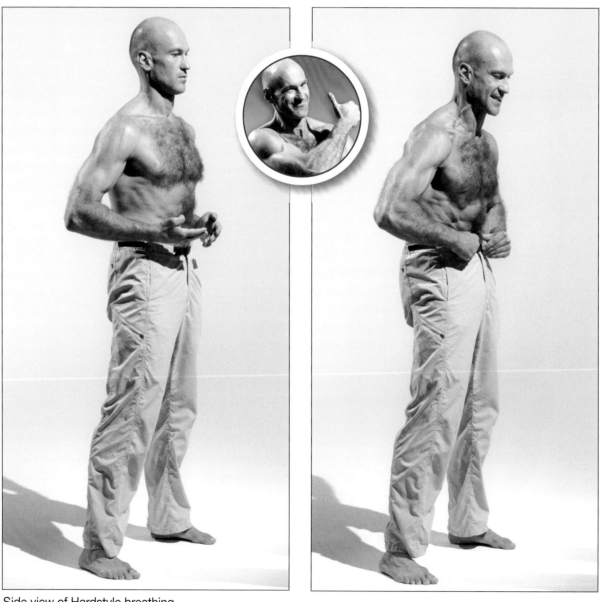

Side view of Hardstyle breathing.

Instead of one long hiss make a series of hisses, each mini-rep progressively ramping up more and more pressure. On a single inhalation. It will probably take 5-10 mini-hisses to empty your lungs but don't bother counting. That was one set.

Over time optimize the number and duration of each mini-hiss to get the most powerful abdominal contraction.

Your spine will naturally flex somewhat as you are blasting your air out. Let flexion happen—but don't make it happen. Full lumbar flexion is unnecessary for maximum abdominal recruitment[15] and the focus on rounding your back takes away from the intensity of the contraction. Listen to Alwyn Cosgrove: "Try to find a crunching motion that creates the most intense pressure on your abdominal muscles with the least movement in your lower back. That's the sweet spot of abdominal training."

Rest for a few minutes before your next set to avoid getting light headed.

In all your Hardstyle drills keep the pressure below your sternum—not in your face, head, or neck. It is a skill. Don't increase the intensity of contraction until you have figured it out.

Keep your shoulders down. Gray Cook has made an insightful observation that many people "use their neck and traps as the core". Don't be one of those.

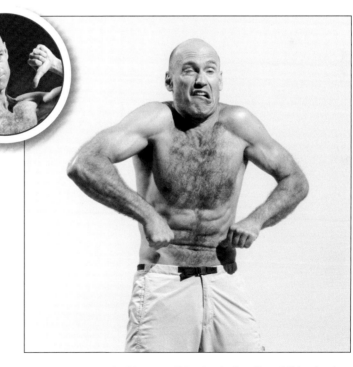

Too much spinal flexion and posterior pelvic tilt!

There are no such things as "Hardstyle face" and "Hardstyle traps"! Knock it off!

Don't rush your Hardstyle breath as this would drop the pressure; it should take you a good five seconds or longer to empty your lungs. And don't purse your lips as if you were in a Pilates class. "Hiss, don't kiss", chuckles Jon Engum, Master RKC and 7th Dan in Taekwondo.

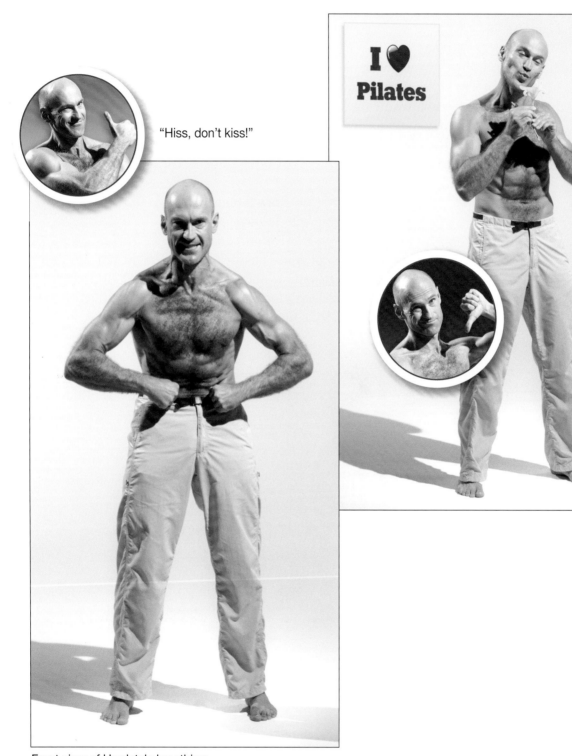

"Hiss, don't kiss!"

I ♥ Pilates

Front view of Hardstyle breathing

On the subject of the depth of your inhalation and exhalation. Victor Popenko, a Russian martial arts strength and conditioning expert, warns, "A person must never have too much or too little air in his lungs." He explains that too much air prevents maximal tensing of the abdominal muscles. Indeed, Russian researchers showed that the greatest strength is achieved when the lungs contain 75% of their vital capacity.[16] Not enough air is just as bad. "When you exhaust your complete breath, a weak spot occurs," warned karate master Kanbun Uechi.

However, since your spine is not under load and hopefully no one is punching you, you may hiss out all of your air when practicing the above Hardstyle breathing drill. You should get a near cramp in your abbies if you do it right. Your waist will naturally shrink as you are squeezing the air out—but don't purposefully pull your stomach in for a beauty queen's fake TVA activation!

On your next set add another Hardstyle subtlety: clench your glutes as well—"pinch a coin".

I cannot overstress how important it is to follow the instructions in this book to the letter! Such subtleties are the essence of the *Hardstyle Abs* program. A seemingly identical exercise performed with a different intention can have a radically different effect. For example, in one study the subjects increased the intensity of the external oblique (EO) contraction by approximately 35% and internal oblique (IO) by approximately 80% when the researchers added a set of specific cues to an abdominal exercise![17]

The resting tension in your abs will increase very quickly. This is great, as long as you do not let the muscles get short. Start stretching and relaxing them between sets. Pick any one of the following exercises.

1. Lie on your back, your legs straight, your head resting on the deck. Gently and rhythmically chop your abs and obliques with the ridges of your hands.

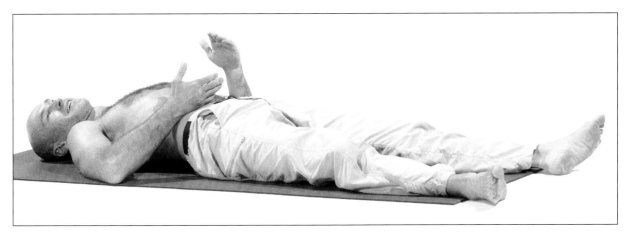

Stretch your arms overhead, and make yourself as long as possible, roll and bend side to side for an extra stretch to your waist.

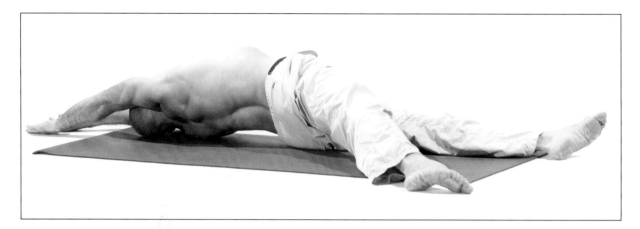

2. The prying cobra. Lie on your stomach with your feet a shoulder's width apart or wider. Plant your hands on the ground, level with your solar plexus. Take a breath, lengthen your spine from head to toe, and push up until your elbows are straight and your shoulders are down. Squeeze your glutes (essential for back safety) and get a big chest. Shift your hips side to side and turn them in order to "pry" the top of the thighs (the hip flexors) and stretch the abs.

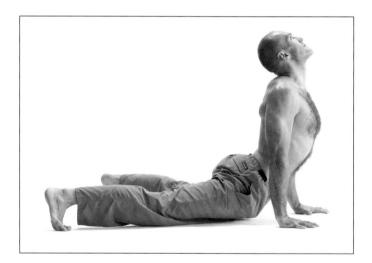

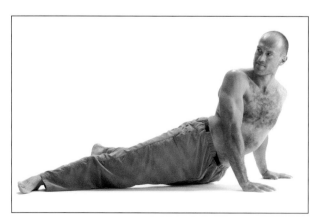
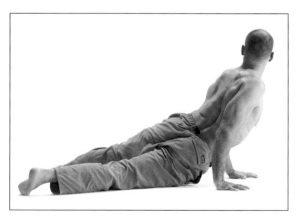

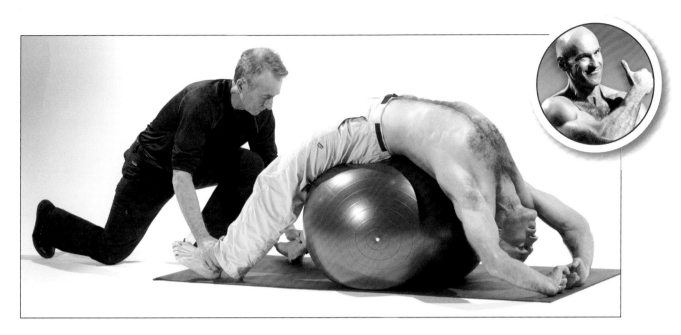

3. Lie on your back on a Swiss ball, your feet hooked under a couch so you can relax and not worry about rolling around. "Lengthen" your spine, stretch your arms, get a big chest, and tighten the glutes. Let your head hang loose. Shift your hips side to side and turn them in order to stretch your midsection and lengthen your spine even more. If necessary, hold on to something for balance. Breathe in a relaxed, passive manner—the opposite of Hardstyle breathing.

To get back up safely place your tongue on the roof of your mouth, squeeze your glutes, and crunch up before sitting up.

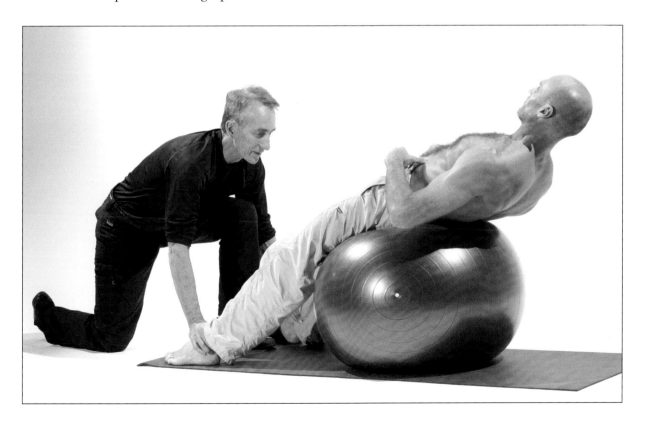

Let us put a finishing touch on the Hardstyle breathing exercise with an ancient technique I call the "karate navel maneuver". The late karate master Masatoshi Nakayama advised: "For strength and stability, it is necessary to have the feeling that the line connecting the navel and the anus is short as possible." It is really another cue to fire up your pelvic floor muscles even more. In addition to contracting the sphincters, the PF muscles tuck in your tailbone, which creates what Prof. Stuart McGill calls "superstiffness".

Initially practice this technique with your knees straight in order not to cheat by performing a posterior pelvic tilt instead.[18] As you are progressing through your Hardstyle breath, bring your tailbone and your navel close together while keeping your legs straight and your kneecaps pulled up. Tense your glutes hard—crush an imaginary walnut—at the same time. Later, once you have understood this subtle movement, you may unlock your knees and add a moderate posterior pelvic tilt to it.

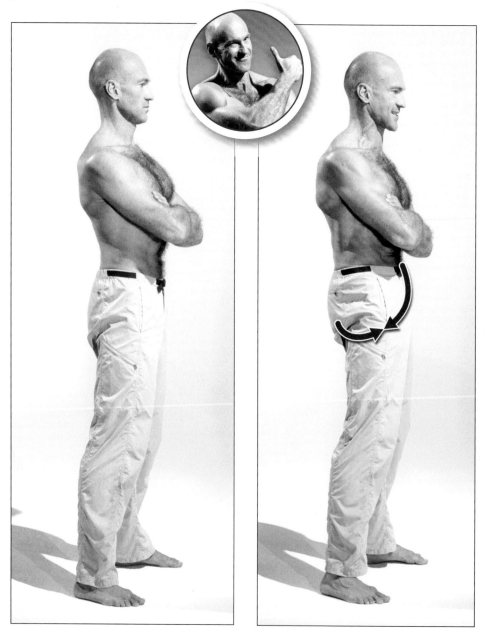

Knees locked.
Pay attention to
how the "karate
navel maneuver"
subtly changes
one's posture in
the second photo.

Not only does the karate navel maneuver give the abs a better workout, it will make you notice-ably stronger in exercises like military presses and pullups. And make your back considerably safer in the former. We use this procedure in many Hardstyle exercises. I must remind you: the effectiveness of the system lies in subtleties like this one.

It is interesting that either loose and weak or tight pelvic floor muscles lead to different health problems, including, surprisingly, orthopedic issues. Strength training must be balanced with stretching. In the case of the PF, deep squats will do the trick.

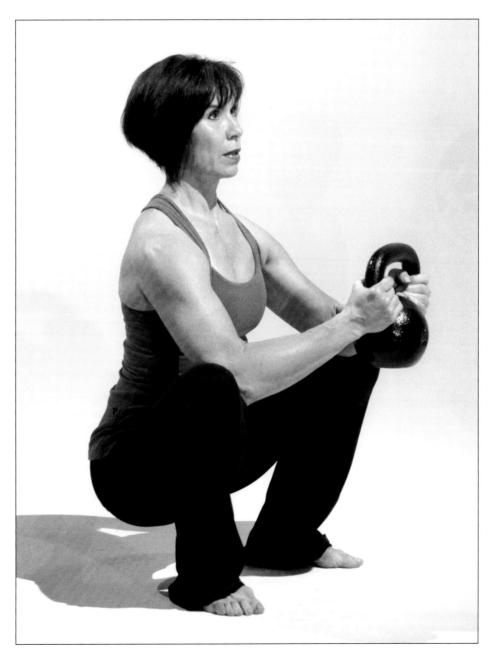

Dan John's goblet squat is a great way to stretch the pelvic floor.

If your hip flexors, the muscles on the top of your thighs that raise your knees, are too tight, you will not be able to perform the karate navel maneuver. Stretch them with the following move and then revisit this powerful karate technique. How do you know if your hip flexors are too tight?— By your posture. Stand up ramrod straight and have someone watch you from the side. If your lower back is very arched and your butt is sticking out, you have this problem. Ditto if you are unable to lock out your knees while standing straight.

I have described several effective hip flexor stretches in my books and DVDs. Here is one more variation recently developed at the RKC school of strength. Assume the kneeling lunge position with your knee very well padded by something like a folded pillow. Do it even if you are a tough guy; knee discomfort will distract you and prevent you from relaxing.

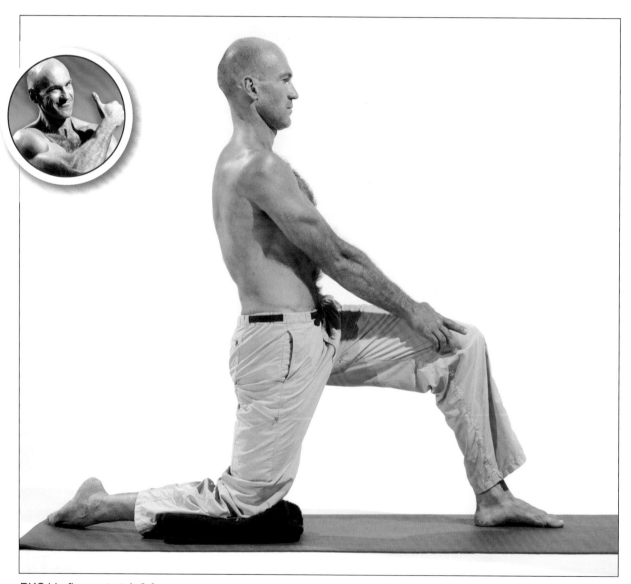

RKC hip flexor stretch 2.0.

Your hips must be square and your torso upright at all times. Your feet and knees should be positioned as they would be if you were to half-kneel wearing cross-country skis and touched a ski with your knee. In other words, nothing should be flopping or twisting away from the planes formed by the "skis". Imagining that you are squeezing something between your knees will help you maintain this alignment.

We are going to start by stretching your right hip flexors, hence your left foot will be in the front. The shin of the front leg should be near vertical; you may have to step forward during the stretch as you are sinking lower and the knee is moving forward.

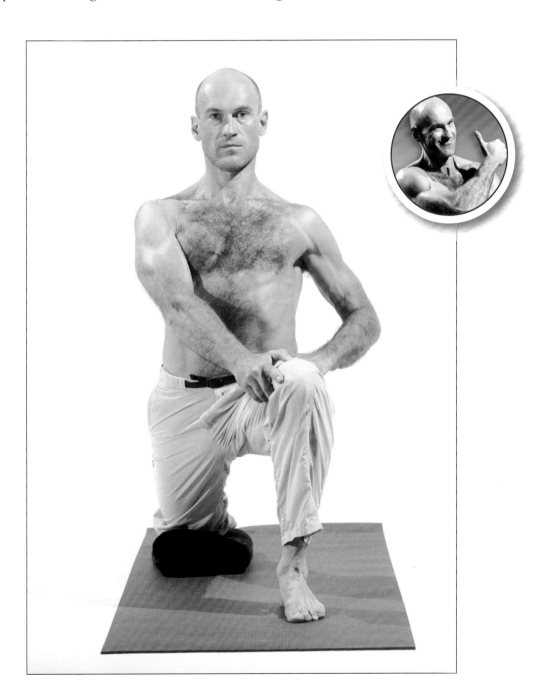

You may hold on to something with your left hand for balance. This object must be on your left and not in the front.

Place your straight arm on the inside of your left knee and push back in order to make your upper back ramrod straight. Raise your chest and head high; Master RKC Dan John would cue you to "be proud of who you are". Your right elbow must stay locked for the duration of the stretch to prevent you from leaning forward and reducing the stretch.

Posteriorly tilt your pelvis: turn your belly button up towards the sky. Maintain this orientation, or at least intention, for the duration of the stretch.

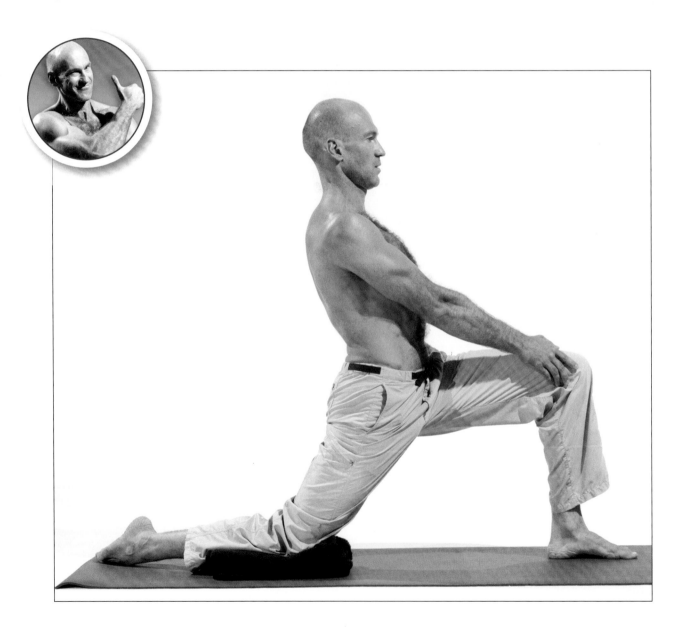

RKC hip flexor stretch 2.0.

Squeeze both glutes and push your pelvis forward. Your pelvis, not your chest! The hips must lead and most of your weight must stay on the rear knee.

You will feel a stretch on the top of the right thigh. Now all you have to do is relax and let your pelvis sink. This requires patience—you need to allow the stretch to happen, not make it happen.

Breathe deeply and slowly. Passively let out all your air with sighs of relief—the opposite of Hardstyle breathing. It helps to visualize breathing out through your tight hip flexors, "breathing the tension out".

Stay down for as long as you can handle it. Stretch each side two to three times almost daily. You may do all your sets back to back, with a couple of minutes of rest, or spread them throughout the day.

Back to our abdominal training with Hardstyle breathing. Here is a variation to give your obliques something extra to worry about. Instead of crunching forward slide your left elbow down lower and lower towards your pelvis, as if a devastating roundhouse kick is coming to your ribs on that side. Maximally shorten the distance between the ribs and the left front corner of the pelvis but don't twist your spine. Do one rep to the left, one to the right, and one to the front.

A word about progression. You can add sets—up to a point. Adding reps is a decidedly bad idea. The amount of tension will be reduced as you fatigue. And subconsciously you will be teaching your body a lesson: "Don't tense so hard, there are many reps ahead, better pace yourself!"

You can make Hardstyle breathing as hard as you want by pressing your tongue harder against your teeth and making a smaller opening. Bernoulli's law decrees that if you reduce the diameter of the opening in half, the resistance to the gas' flow will increase fourfold.

Practice Hardstyle breathing almost every day, throughout the day, for instance a set every hour. One can easily recover from this type of exercise, so it will not take anything away from your sports and strength training. Make

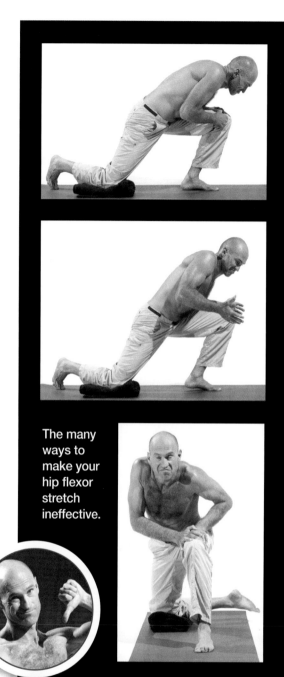

The many ways to make your hip flexor stretch ineffective.

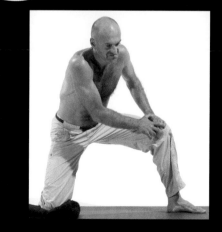

each rep as concentrated as possible and don't forget to take long breaks between sets in order not to get lightheaded. Keep the pressure in your stomach and away from your neck, face, and head. Stretch your abs after every set.

Do not do any other direct abdominal training—I insist. You may continue your strength training as usual.

Eat as a Russian noble or an officer in Imperial Russia's officers' corps. As described by Leo Tolstoy in **Anna Karenina** in the late XIX century:

> *Vronsky came to the regimental mess for his beefsteak earlier than usual. There was no need for him to follow strict training, since his weight came in just under the regulation hundred-sixty pounds; but he had to avoid getting fat too, and he avoided sweet and starchy food.*

In the end of two weeks you should see a very noticeable difference in your "dear abbies". Before moving on to the next phase please drop me a note on the www.DragonDoor.com forum and let me know how well you are doing.

FOOTNOTES

8   Zatsiorsky (1995)

9   Zatsiorsky (1995). In some Russian sources, e.g. Ilyin (2003), it is referred to as the *viscero-motor reflex*.

10 "IAP increases during muscular efforts, especially during a Valsalva maneuver. As a result of internal support [from increase IAP], the pressure on intervertebral discs can be reduced by up to 20% on average and up to 40% in extreme cases. Internal support of the spinal column can be compared to the mechanical action of a ball located in the abdominal cavity." (Zatsiorsky, 1995)

11 Floyd & Walls (1953), Cardus et al (1963), Scott et al. (1964). These and several other references to Western research in these footnotes can be traced to Basmaijan, JV and De Luca, CJ. *Muscles Alive: Their Functions Revealed by Electromyography* (5th ed.). Baltimore: Williams & Wilkins, 1985.

12 Sapsford et al. (2001)

13 Bors & Blinn (1965)

14 The "Darth Vader breath" of the kind used in the study cited by Zatsiorsky (1995) appears to be more appropriate when one is practicing stabilizing a neutral spine, as in the plank. It is not used in *Hardstyle Abs* because it does not recruit the rectus abdominis sufficiently.

15 Sarti et al. (1996)

16 Seropegin (1965)

17 Karst & Willett (2001)

18 The technical name for what we are doing is "counternutation of the sacrum". This means your "tail tucks in" underneath the pelvis. Do not confuse it with a posterior pelvic tilt, which is a grosser movement—tipping the whole "bowl" of the pelvis back. While helpful in promoting a stronger abdominal contraction, at this point a posterior pelvic tilt would just distract you from a much subtler sacral counternutation.

The Hardstyle Sit-up:
how to defeat your hip flexors and make your abs rule

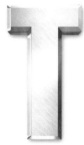

The hip flexors just cannot help meddling in the abs' business.

The rectus or "six-pack" connects your pubic bone to your breastbone. When this muscle contracts, it pulls your pelvis and rib cage together, rounding your back in the process, as in a crunch. This is called "forward spinal flexion".

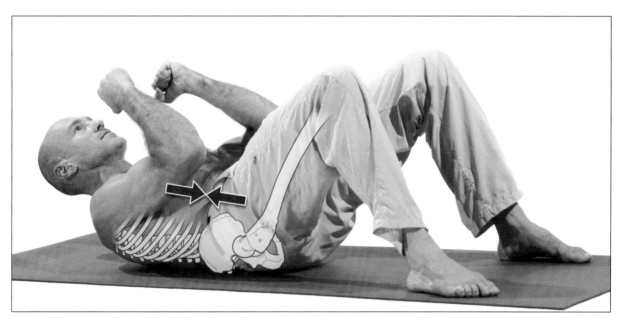

Forward spinal flexion.

The psoas major originates on the vertebrae of the lower back, and inserts into the top of the thighbone. When this muscle contracts, it jackknifes the body. When you do a sit-up, you literally pull yourself up by your lumbar spine, which can lead to back problems or aggravate existing ones.

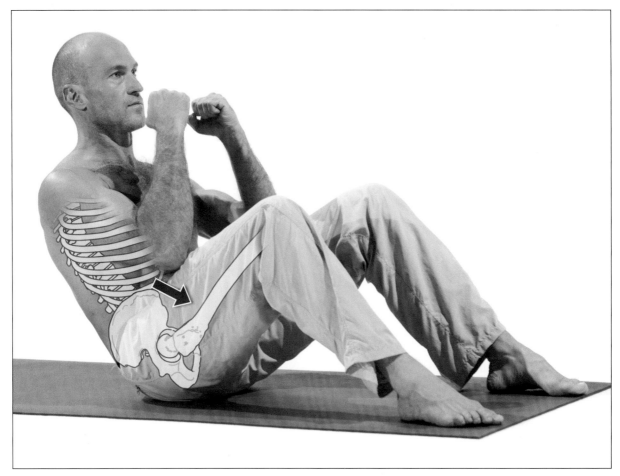

When you do a sit-up, you literally pull yourself up by your lumbar spine.

(The following naïve view is common among the new breed of trainees "enlightened" to embrace integration as opposed to isolation: "I want all of my muscles strong, the psoas as well as the abs!" Fine, but you have to earn the right to strengthen your psoas by making your abs strong enough to balance out its pull. I am not against a strong psoas; I am for balanced strength development.)

Until the recent plank fashion, the "solution" was to avoid hip flexion, or sit-ups, and do only spinal flexion, or crunches. Because there is no hip flexion in the crunch, it supposedly did not involve the psoas and gave the lower back a break. You wish.

Clinicians determined that it is impossible to completely eliminate the hip flexor recruitment during a crunch.[19] This is especially true for people with faulty movement patterns and weak abs. A person with weak abdominals relies on his or her stronger hip flexors even during crunches. The trainee cannot get his torso off the floor by rounding his back with his abs, so he compensates by yanking on his spine with his hip flexors to gain momentum! It does not take a rocket scientist to figure out that such training is worthless for the abs and dangerous to the spine. (And even if the person has healthy movement patterns and uses his abs correctly and his hip flexors minimally, the crunch will not allow him to generate enough tension to make it an effective exercise unless he has an exceptional "mind to muscle connection".)

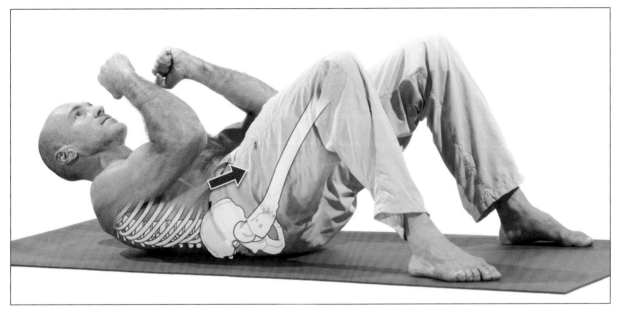

A weak and/or uncoordinated Comrade will yank on his spine with his psoas even during crunches.

The problem of the hip flexor involvement was radically solved by Vladimir Janda, M.D., from Czech Republic, the consultant on rehabilitation for the World Health Organization and one of the world's leading experts on back problems, muscle function analysis and evaluation. Professor Janda relaxed the psoas using the neurological phenomenon of *reciprocal inhibition*. When a muscle contracts, its antagonist, or the opposite number, relaxes. It is about efficiency. The alternative would be similar to stepping on the gas and the brake simultaneously.

Dr. Janda redesigned the sit-up in such a manner that the hip extensor muscles, the hamstrings and the glutes, were activated. Reciprocal inhibition took place and the hip flexors relaxed. The result: back stress was eliminated and the abdominals were "isolated"! The exercise was excruciatingly hard; Joseph Horrigan, D.C. mentions that a number of Olympians struggled to complete even a couple of reps.

I have made modifications to the original. Enter the Hardstyle sit-up.

Why I Modified the Original Janda Sit-Up

If you are not a nerd, don't read this.

The Czech doctor had his patient assume the standard bent knee sit-up/crunch position, placed his hands under the latter's calves, and gently pulled up. The patient attempted to crunch up while digging his heels into the ground and pushing the balls of the feet downward against the doc's knees—an isometric calf raise.

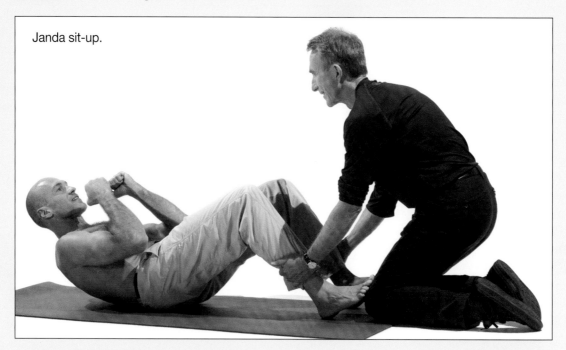

Janda sit-up.

The purpose of digging the heels in was obvious—to recruit the hip extensors and thus inhibit the hip flexors. The toe pushing business was supposed to enhance this process by setting off a muscle synergy present in walking. Or at least so the story went. A later study discovered that Janda sit-ups recruited the hip flexors even more than regular sit-ups…[20]

Here is what I think went down. The subjects were instructed to pull their feet towards their butts to activate the hamstrings. We know that the hams' two primary functions are hip extension and knee flexion. Which one do you think they were exercising when they were pulling their heels towards their tails?—It had to be the knee flexion. And the hip action synergistic to it is also flexion.

I can also see how someone who followed Dr. Janda's original instructions could have gone wrong and pushed up instead of down with the balls of their feet and wedged their heels to formally fulfill the heels down command. The exercise would have practically turned into a conventional feet anchored sit-up.

Whether I am right or not, I have made some changes to Janda's original sit-up to foolproof it. I called the exercise the "modified Janda situp" and took flak from some medical professionals familiar with the late doctor's work. They argued that there was not a lot of Janda left in the exercise. Hence, from now on it is the "Hardstyle sit-up".

My version calls for sitting up all the way. I had expected it to lead to a greater abdominal activation than from just a crunch, as we later confirmed at Prof. Stuart McGill's lab. A possible explanation: "The hip flexion phase [of a sit-up] provides strong resistance against the abdominals. The hip flexors pull strongly downward on the pelvis as the abdominals work to hold the trunk in flexion and the pelvis in the direction of the posterior tilt."[21]

Obviously, a full sit-up cannot be done without the hip flexors. But whatever the physiological mechanism, the Hardstyle sit-up has a remarkable record of building rock hard abs and making backs feel great. Either the hip flexors are not pulling as hard as usual or, more likely, the abs are contracting much harder and balancing out their pull against the spine; whatever it is, it works.

A powerful contraction of the glutes is likely to be giving the back a break.[22] And here is another possible mechanism that brings some people with back pain relief when they hit Hardstyle sit-ups. Patients with chronic back pain have difficulty recruiting the internal obliques.[23] Research shows that exercises strengthening the IO help people with back pain because of these muscles' role in stabilizing the spine.[24] Our measurements at Prof. McGill's lab showed peak recruitment of the IO reach 100% maximal voluntary contraction (MVC) during Hardstyle sit-ups. Perhaps this exercise wakes up this muscle in folks with a dysfunctional firing pattern?

Whatever the mechanism, Hardstyle sit-ups deliver.

"MY CHIROPRACTOR TOLD ME THAT I SHOULD BUY THIS [DEVICE] AND STOP DOING SIT-UPS. I HAVE BEEN USING THE AB PAVELIZER FOR 2 WEEKS (EVERY OTHER DAY) AND MY BACK PAIN IS GONE. I AM ALSO STARTING DOING THE BACK STRETCHING EXERCISES THAT WERE INCLUDING IN THE PACKAGING AT THE SAME TIME. ACCORDING TO MY CHIROPRACTOR IT IS BOTH OF THEM THAT ARE HELPING ME. SO I WILL STAY WITH IT."

—MARK HILBURGER, UECHI-RYU KARATE PRACTITIONER

"I AM 56 YEARS OLD... I HAVE FOUND THAT, OVER THE YEARS, ANYTIME I HAVE EXPERIENCED BACK PAIN, I DUST OFF THE AB PAVELIZER, HIT A FEW SESSIONS AND THE PAIN IS GONE. MY AB STRENGTH FEELS GREAT. "
—ROB DREWRY, MICHIGAN

But first, let us stretch your lower back (provided you are not flexion intolerant). Dr. Janda observed that some of his patients felt back tightness during the abdominal exercise and stretching took care of it.

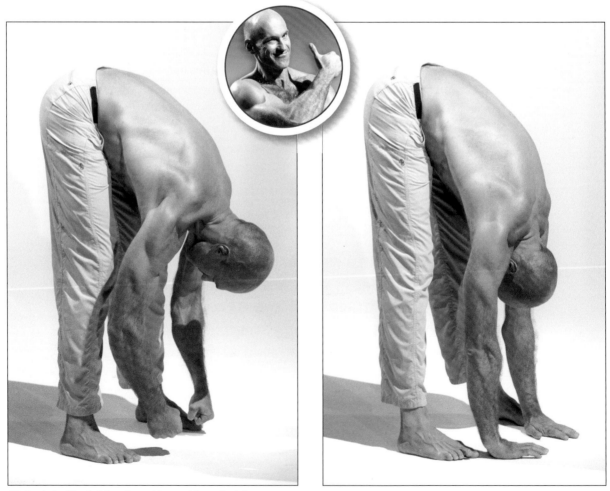

Relax into Stretch back and hamstring stretch.

Always stretch barefoot. Keeping your knees nearly locked, slowly bend over as far as you can. Relax your head, don't hold it up. Look at some spot behind your knees, not between your feet.

Inhale, grip the ground with your toes, and tighten up the muscles on the rear side of your body: your back, glutes, and hamstrings. Imagine your body is a tightly clenched fist. Indeed, clenching your fists will help.

Hold the tension—and your breath—for a second, then suddenly relax and let the air out with tension. You will drop an inch or two increasing your stretch. I like the graphic description of this tension/release sequence by Dr. Judd Biasiotto: "You must relax instantly... picture yourself exerting all your strength in an effort to push a large boulder off a sheer cliff. When suddenly the boulder goes over the edge, there is no active resistance to your pushing and all your straining instantly ceases. It is that feeling, that nothingness after the boulder drops, that you are striving to obtain when you "turn off your source of power".

Sigh with relief, and repeat. Make sure not to decrease the stretch when you are tensing and inhaling—stay at the same level.

When you can no longer increase the range of motion, bend your knees, and stand up tensing your glutes. Bending your knees on the way up is essential for your back safety.

Are you ready for the Hardstyle sit-up? Although it looks innocent, it is shockingly tough. Like the bodyguards of the Soviet leaders: regular looking guys without bull's necks, enlarged knuckles, or scars. They wore nice suits and knew how to use fancy silverware at a state reception. Behind harmless and inconspicuous exteriors hid deadly skills.

The Hardstyle sit-up demands a training partner or some hardware. Let us start with the partner version. Assume the top of the standard bent knee sit-up position, your knees at a ninety-degree angle and your feet flat. Ask your training partner to pull on the very middle of your calves with a towel. He will be tempted to use his hands; do not let him as this will allow him to unconsciously help you cheat! Tell him to pull up at a forty-five degree angle. Ten pounds of force will do in the beginning. You will optimize it later. Do not wear clothes which would slide easily on the surface on which you are exercising. None of that sissy Lycra.

Russian research demonstrated that an eccentric contraction followed by an isometric contraction produced the greatest muscle tension[25]. So you will start your Hardstyle sit-up from the top down. EMG studies by UCLA professor Dr. Laurence Morehouse, who designed strength and conditioning programs for NASA astronauts, confirmed that this applies to abdominal activation in sit-ups.

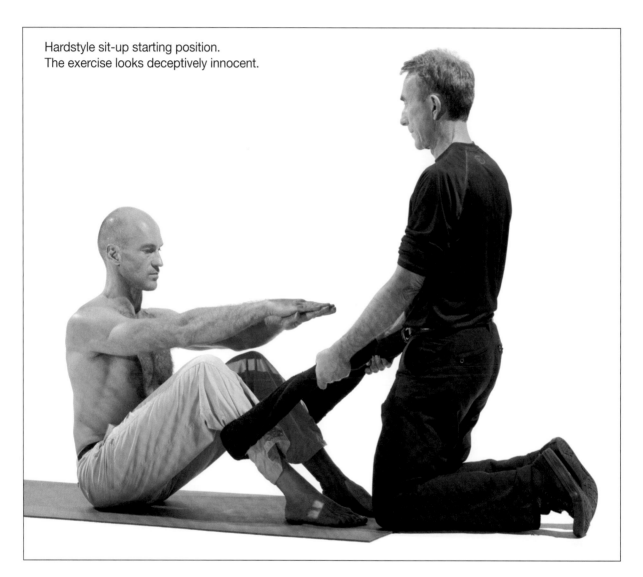

Hardstyle sit-up starting position.
The exercise looks deceptively innocent.

On the top of the Hardstyle sit-up your lower back should be slightly flexed and your pelvis slightly tucked in. Slightly—do not force either. Inhale, perform the karate navel maneuver, tense your glutes, and press your feet down into the deck. Hardstyle breathe in a familiar series of sharp hisses until you have emptied most of your air and got a nice cramp in the abbies. Your final hiss should be as sharp as a cough[26] or a karateka's "Kiai!" Dan John half jokingly says that there is no better ab work then vomiting. Strive for that feeling—without the help of undercooked chicken.

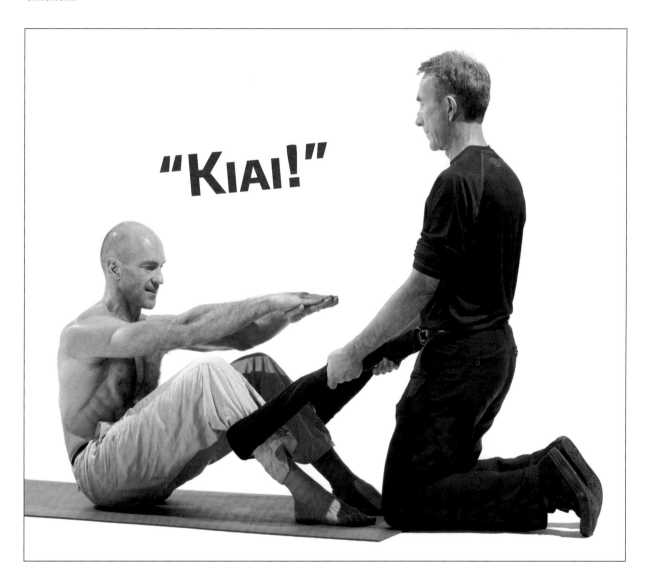

To get an even greater contraction, use the following technique.[27] Reach your hands forward and place one hand on top of the other. Keeping your shoulders down press the hands hard against each other (if you understand how to externally rotate your shoulders and depress your scapulae, do that too). This will stiffen your lats and light up your whole midsection. Don't reach forward by rounding your shoulders (you will be tempted to when the going gets tough). You will discover that you have to use various upper back muscles to keep your shoulders in line.

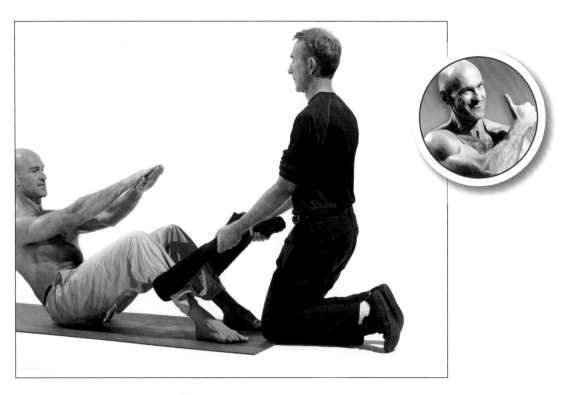

Don't reach forward by rounding your shoulders when the going gets tough. Use your upper back muscles to keep your shoulders in line.

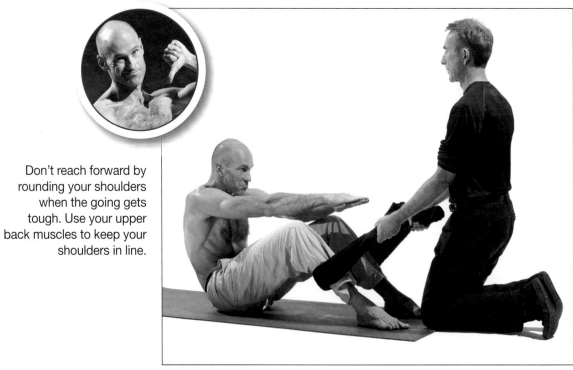

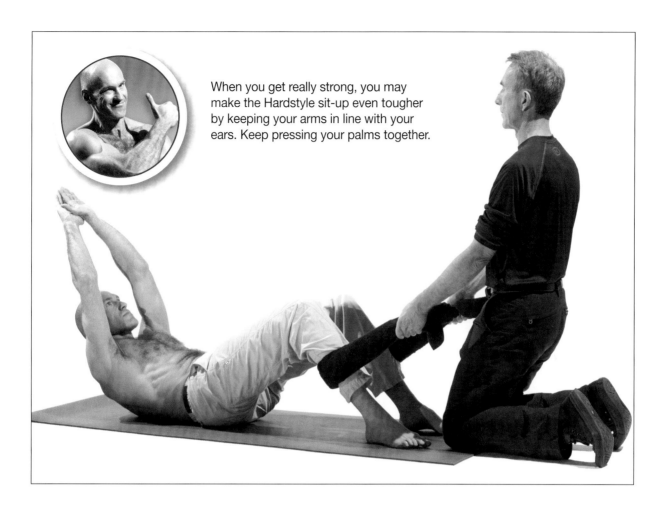

When you get really strong, you may make the Hardstyle sit-up even tougher by keeping your arms in line with your ears. Keep pressing your palms together.

Lie back slowly. I will qualify what "slowly" means. Not an exaggerated ten second negative, just slow enough to eliminate all momentum and maximize tension. If you are strong enough to get all the way down to the deck, it takes approximately three seconds—the same time as it would naturally take you to go back up in a very challenging repetition. In Hardstyle strength training we move the way one moves under a very heavy load—with the unrushed confidence of a tow truck, not exaggerated slowness. Avoid the following bad habit: hitting a sticking point about halfway down and, fearful of going deeper, just hanging there forever, and then collapsing. This is not the Hardstyle way.

So lie back moderately slowly without losing any abdominal and glute tension. "Sniff" or, as the late Dr. Mel Siff used to teach, "sip" air, but do not breathe deep as this would make the contraction weaker. "Breathe behind the shield", as they say in some karate styles. Deep breathing makes muscle tension drop and holding your breath under tension for an extended period of time is unhealthy. "Breathing behind the shield" is a useful compromise. As always, keep your face impassive, your neck and traps relaxed. You will not be able to totally relax them but do your best.

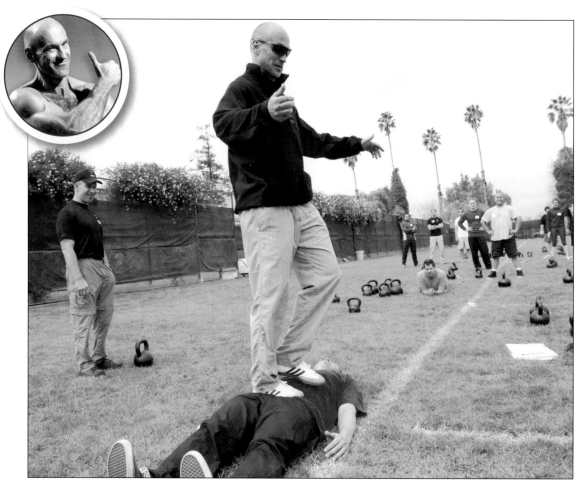

Here is how we teach "breathing behind the shield" at RKC kettlebell instructor courses.

Keep digging your heels down into the ground against your partner's towel pull. Your feet may neither come up nor drag closer towards your butt—either would indicate cheating with your hip flexors. Ditto if your body is sliding towards your feet. Keep cramping those glutes!

When you have reached the depth where you cannot continue downward without letting your abs and/or glutes go slack, pause for a moment, and slowly power back up. Don't jerk! On the way up keep "breathing behind the shield". When you have reached the top, perform the familiar series of Hardstyle hisses until you have explosively emptied your lungs.

Russian research[28] showed that the ability to store and reuse the tension loaded into the muscles in the yielding phase of the movement separates elite athletes from the "also-rans". Visualize your abdominals as rubber bands. As you stretch them on descent, load them with elastic tension. The following quote from Prof. Stuart McGill, although taken out of context, should drive the point home: "The abdominal wall functions like a spring and should be trained that way."

Do 3-5 reps, then rest for 3-5min.

Lie back slowly.

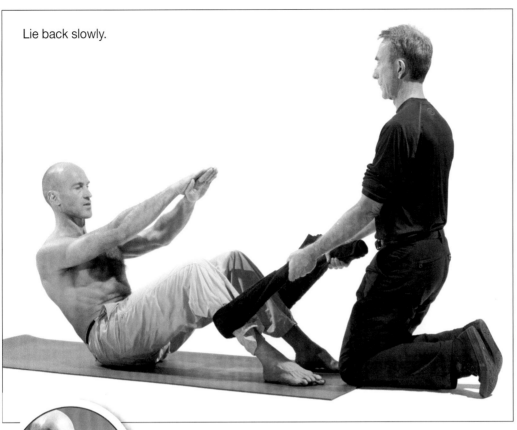

Reverse the movement before you
lose tension and collapse.

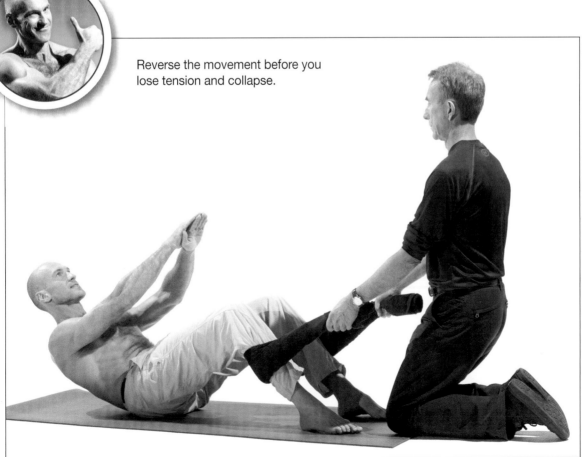

One more time: keep cramping your glutes, don't release them for a moment.

If your calves cramp, ignore them. Provided you are well hydrated and your electrolytes are where they need to be, they will adapt in a few sessions.

On your next set add a subtlety that will make the drill more neck friendly. Use Stuart McGill's imagery and "picture the head and neck as a rigid block on the thoracic spine". In other words, from your sternum up you are an insect, with no mobility whatsoever! In reality, you will not be able to avoid all movement in the area, just do your best.

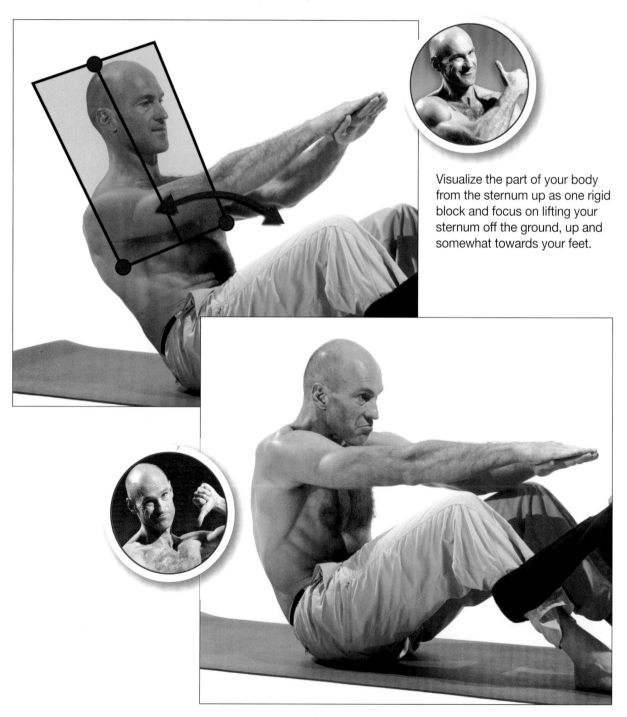

Visualize the part of your body from the sternum up as one rigid block and focus on lifting your sternum off the ground, up and somewhat towards your feet.

Start by saying farewell to the common practice of initiating a sit-up by tucking in your chin and curling up your upper back. Then tell yourself that you are not a chicken and swear off from jutting your chin forward as well. Visualize the part of your body from the sternum up as one rigid block and focus on lifting your sternum off the ground, up and somewhat towards your feet.

Once more: the focus is on lifting the sternum. Although your neck will not budge, shoot your eyes down between your feet; this will reflexively amplify the abdominals' contraction. Keep contracting your glutes. Learn to fire your glutes and abs as one muscle—this is one of the secrets of gymnasts' upper body strength.

You might ask: what should the pelvis and lower back do?—If you follow the instructions and cramp your "cheeks", keep your feet in place, and move with confident slowness, this area will take care of itself. Your spine will flex and your pelvis will tuck in or tilt posteriorly—just the right amount. Eventually, as you get more coordinated, your glutes and the pelvis will feel like a smoothly rolling, fully pumped up tire.

Do not force either the flexion or the tilt! Remember Cosgrove.

The Role of the Posterior Pelvic Tilt and Spinal Flexion in Abdominal Training

I am warning you: this is boring stuff. Feel free to skip it and do another set of Hardstyle sit-ups instead.

Just to make sure that we are on the same page, the "neutral" pelvis refers to the position it is in when you are standing upright. If you think of the pelvis as a bowl and then tilt it and dump some soup onto the front of your pants, you have an anterior tilt. If the soup spills into your back pockets, the tilt is posterior.

Leading sports scientists Drs. Verkhoshansky and Siff explain:

> *The pelvis plays a vital role in the ability of the athlete to produce strength efficiently and safely, because it is the major link between the spinal column and the lower extremities... a **neutral pelvic tilt** offers the least stressful position for sitting, standing and walking. It is only when a load (or bodymass) is lifted or resisted that other types of pelvic tilt become necessary. Even then, only sufficient tilt is used to prevent excessive spinal flexion or extension... The **posterior pelvic tilt** is the appropriate pelvic rotation for sit-ups or lifting objects above waist level. Conversely... the anterior pelvic tilt is the correct pelvic rotation for squatting [and] lifting heavy loads off the floor".[29]

Pelvic Tilts

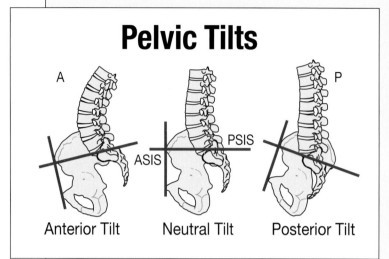

A

ASIS

PSIS

P

Anterior Tilt   Neutral Tilt   Posterior Tilt

Translation: generally you want to do with your spine and pelvis the opposite of what the load wants them to do. When you are picking up heavy iron off the platform, the barbell wants your back to round and your pelvis to tilt posteriorly. Hence weightlifting coaches keep barking at their athletes to arch and lift their tails. On the other hand, when you are doing a handstand, sit-ups, or any other abdominal exercise involving hip flexion, your spine is determined to go into hyperextension and your pelvis wants to tip anteriorly. This is why gymnastics coaches yell at their charges to tuck in their tails and fight the "banana" shaped arched handstands every bit as ruthlessly as their weightlifting colleagues fight round back cleans. Gymnasts also use this alignment—a posterior pelvic tilt with a maximal abdominal and gluteal tension—in a great many strength maneuvers like the iron cross. Because this so-called "hollow position" (see the photo) makes them super-strong. (The hollow position has nothing to do with TVA hollowing, by the way!)

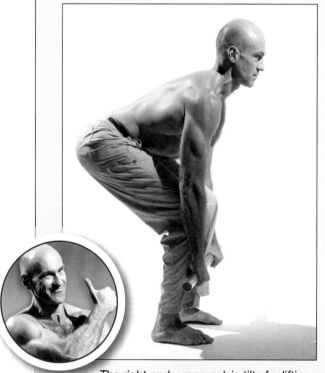

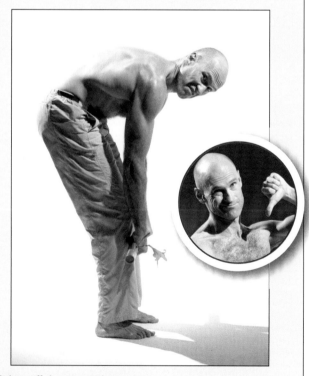

The right and wrong pelvic tilts for lifting weights off the ground.

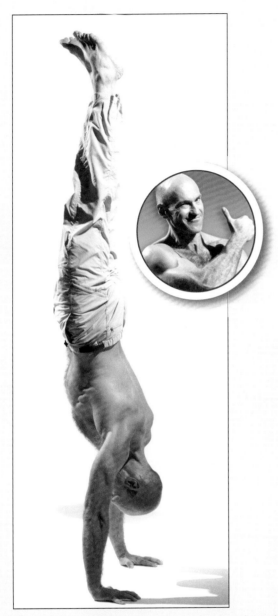
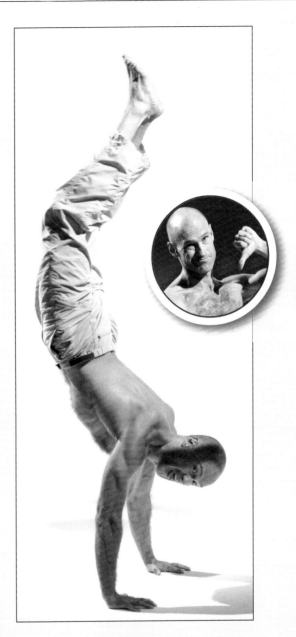

The right and wrong pelvic tilts for the handstand.

It must be noted that while these weightlifting and gymnastic maneuvers greatly improve strength and safety in their respective disciplines, you should not "live in your sports posture", as Master RKC Mark Reifkind warns us. If your training molds your body in such a way that you start walking around with a big arch in your lower back and your tail perking up—as many Americans, couch potatoes and athletes alike, do—you are going to be a hurting unit. Elite sprint coach Barry Ross reveals the mystery of the ever-popular hamstring pull: "The anterior pelvis

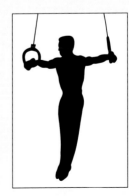

tilt can cause irritation to the sciatic nerve as well as hamstring strains or tears. Coaches and athletes often believe that sore hamstrings are the product of lack of stretching, when in fact the hammies are being hammered by the effects of an anterior pelvic tilt. Well-developed abdominal muscles are a necessity to correct the problem." Add back problems to the list of the joys of living in an anterior pelvic tilt.

Corrective work for this condition includes strengthening the abs and the external obliques, waking up the glutes, and stretching the back muscles and the hip flexors. The *Hardstyle Abs* plan covers all of the above and your doc is very likely to give it two thumbs up. It is worth noting that 85% of men and 75% of women live with an anterior pelvic tilt![30]

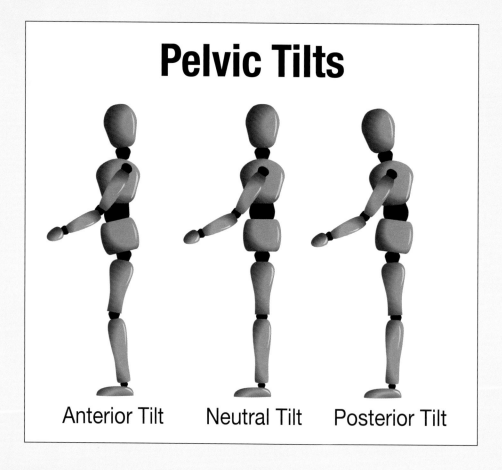

Pelvic Tilts

Anterior Tilt   Neutral Tilt   Posterior Tilt

If, on the other hand, your genes and life have given you a posterior pelvic tilt—6% of men and 7% of women[31]—and a flat spine, you should hold off the *Hardstyle Abs* plan until you have addressed your condition with a professionally designed corrective exercise plan. Once you are back to plumb, a balanced training program, which involves Hardstyle kettlebells, is in order.

Living with a posterior tilt and a flat spine is not a dream either, because prolonged flexion sets one up for various back and neck problems. But you have to go into this position briefly if you are to train your abbies to the max. Full disclosure: world's top spine biomechanist Prof. Stuart McGill is not a fan of spinal flex-ion. According to his research, this is a common lower back injury mechanism, which is why his torso training prescriptions involve only exercises with an immobilized neutral spine. If you are what specialists call "flexion intolerant", the *Hardstyle Abs* plan, with a possible exception of Hardstyle breathing, probably is not for you. Get McGill's classic *Ultimate Back Fitness and Performance* from **www.backfitpro.com** and follow the good doctor's lead.

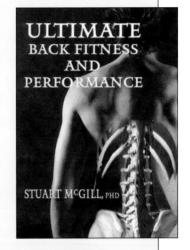

McGill acknowledges that everyone has different levels of spine flexion tolerance.[32] If you can take it and want world-class abs, read on.

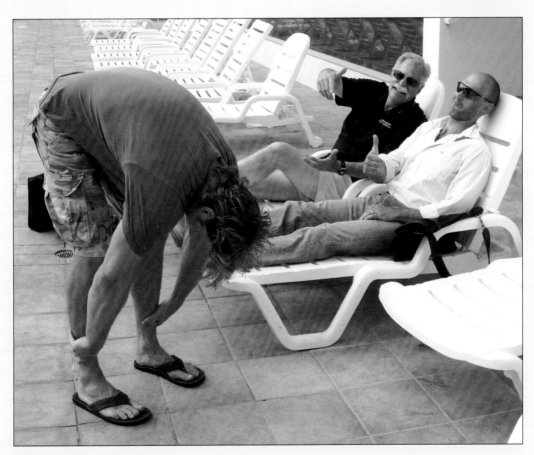

Chad Waterbury demonstrating the type of spine flexion to avoid to Stuart and Pavel.
Photo courtesy Chad Waterbury

This is a good time to explain why spine flexion and posterior pelvic tilting are present in *Hardstyle Abs.*

There are at least three reasons to flex the spine if you are to build the strongest abs.

First, Russian scientists, while endorsing isometric training, have concluded that you will not reach your strength potential if you use it exclusively. A combination of holding, lifting, and lowering is called for.[33]

Second, one of the goals of the *Hardstyle Abs* program is myofibrillar hypertrophy of the midsection muscles. Research and experience show that isometric training is an inferior modality for building muscle.

Third, for all their pretty boy side effects, the *Hardstyle Abs'* primary goal is strength. Strength is tension. In my coaching experience, one cannot achieve the greatest level of tension without shortening the muscle. And when the abs and the external obliques shorten, the spine flexes and the pelvis tilts posteriorly. Indeed, the posterior pelvic tilt has a very powerful effect on activating the abs.[34] To give you an idea, the rectus abdominis were clocked as being 57% more active with a posterior pelvic tilt than an anterior tilt, with a neutral pelvis being in the middle.[35] (In the rectus femoris, a hip flexor muscle, the order was predictably the opposite.[36]) A posterior pelvic tilt elicits a greater activity in the lower abs than spine flexion.[37] Emphasizing spinal flexion recruits the upper abs more and emphasizing the posterior pelvic tilt lights up the lower abs more.[38] Both are present in the Hardstyle sit-up.

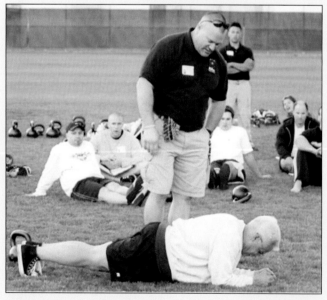

Even if your sport does not demand spinal flexion, once you have trained your abs in flexion—properly, the Hardstyle way—they will be able to generate a lot more tension even with a neutral spine. After a few months of *Hardstyle Abs* try the plank and you will be blown away by the amount of tension you can generate. And you will be able to hold the neutral posture much better.

USAPL National Champion and IPF Powerlifting Team USA Head Coach Dr. Michael Hartle, Senior RKC is kicking Masters' IPF World Champion Doug Dienelt, RKC to test the latter's plank.

Stretch your "dear abbies", rest for 3-5min—no less!—and do another set. 3-5 sets of 3-5 reps with 3-5min of rest is a standard Hardstyle strength practice. Do this three times a week.

Eventually—if you remember to keep your glutes tight!—you should reach the point where your shoulder blades and the back of the head brush the floor. Congratulations! But this should not stop you from occasionally doing the easier version of your early Hardstyle days—top half reps—for a change of pace and a greater contraction. You may also use the "1½" technique alternating half reps and full reps: down halfway, up all the way, down all the way, up all the way, etc.

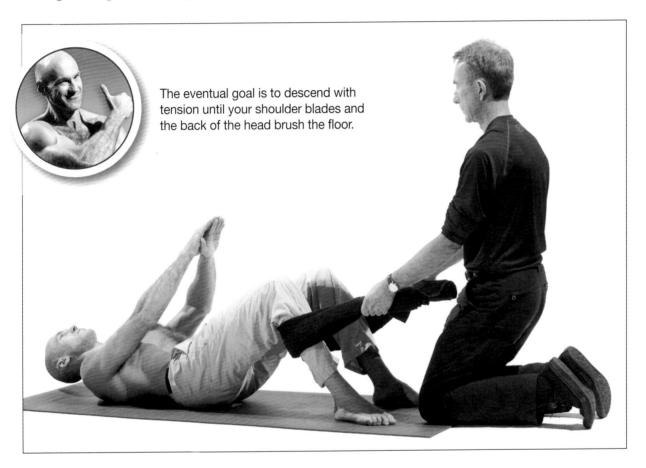

The eventual goal is to descend with tension until your shoulder blades and the back of the head brush the floor.

At some point you should add a tougher Hardstyle sit-up variation, which has you start your reps on the bottom. From a relaxed supine position fire your glutes and abs, pressurize, and come up under control, as usual. Blow out your air on the top, get a good abdominal cramp, and head down "sniffing" air a little. When your scapulae and the back of your head touch the ground, let out a sigh of relief and relax completely for a second or more. Then take a breath, reengage the tension, and continue. As we will see later, this practice of creating tension out of nothing is very valuable in your strength practice, which is why it is present in the methodologies of elite strength coaches like Marty Gallagher.

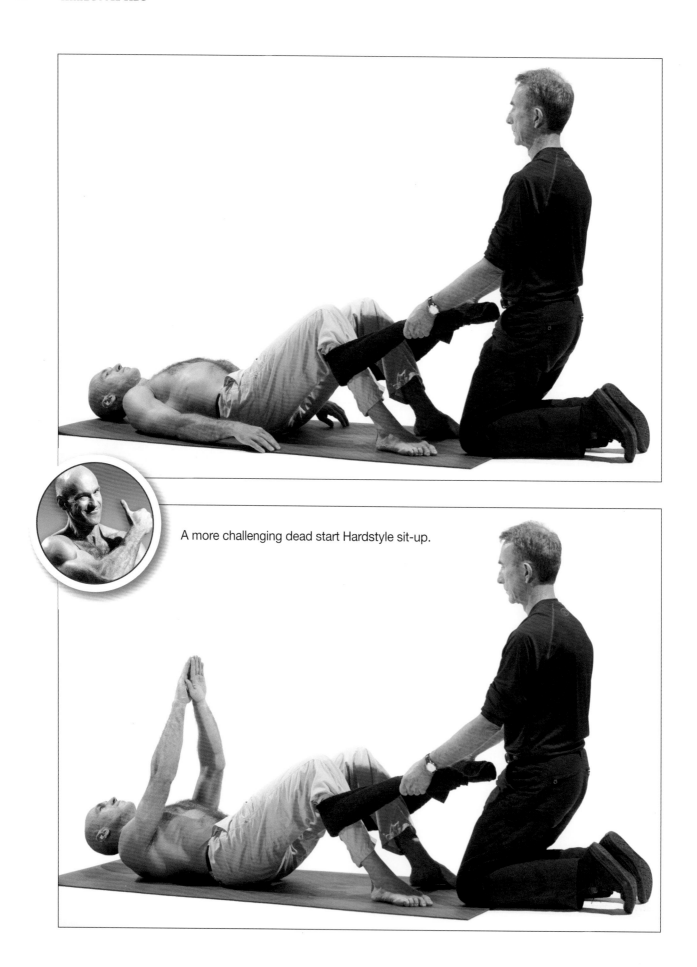

A more challenging dead start Hardstyle sit-up.

Just in case you don't have a handy training partner, I designed the trusty **Ab Pavelizer™** (US **Patent No. 6,991,591 B1**). Please do not take this as a sales pitch: the Pavelizer works a lot better than a human.

Place your Ab Pavelizer™ on a high friction surface, e.g. a yoga mat. Slap on a barbell plate—10 pounds is a good start—and sit on the ground in front of this deceptively innocent looking device. Spin on your butt and place your calves on top of the roller pads. Press down until your feet are on the deck.

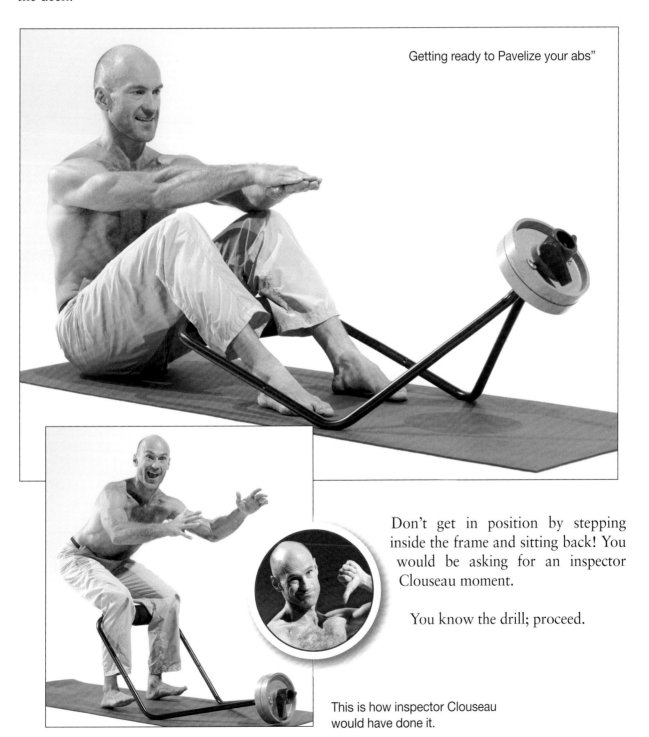

Getting ready to Pavelize your abs"

Don't get in position by stepping inside the frame and sitting back! You would be asking for an inspector Clouseau moment.

You know the drill; proceed.

This is how inspector Clouseau would have done it.

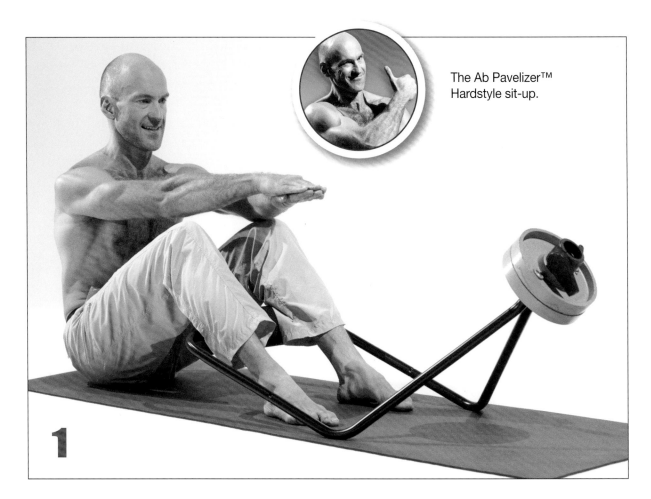

The Ab Pavelizer™
Hardstyle sit-up.

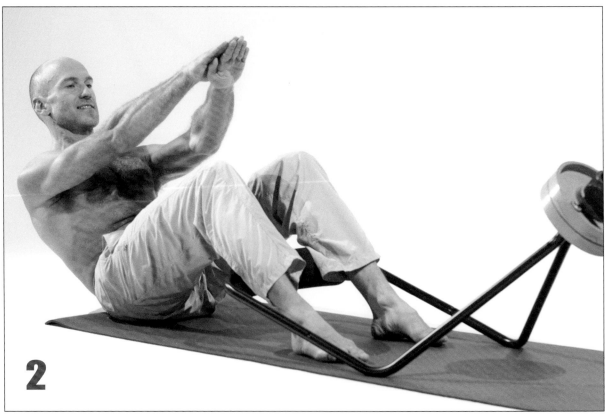

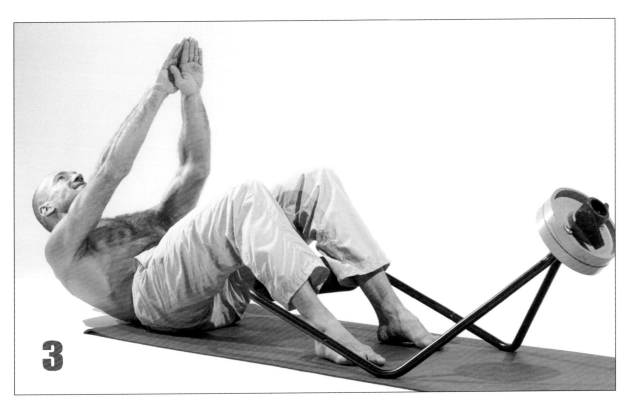

The device provides two types of feedback warning that you are doing the exercise wrong. You could get tricky and try to use your hip flexors by pulling your knees towards your chest. But the moment you do, the Ab Pavelizer™ will slide across the floor towards you. Sirens go off, guns are drawn, you know you had better get your act together!

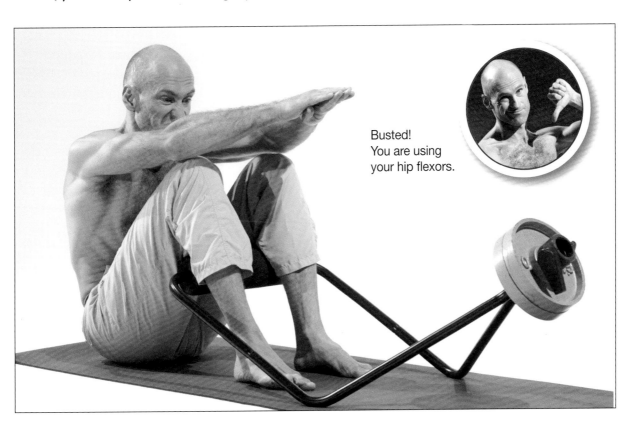

Busted!
You are using
your hip flexors.

And if you relax your butt muscles even for a moment, the Ab Pavelizer™ that never sleeps will lift your feet right off the floor. Sirens, guns, and the whole unpleasant thing again. So you had better get it right!

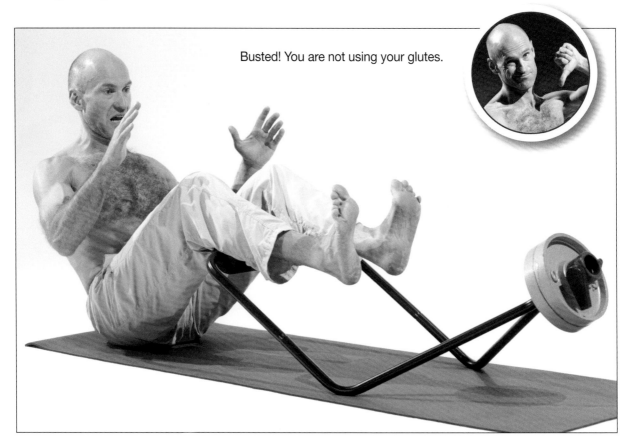

Busted! You are not using your glutes.

Progress to the point where you are using 25 pounds if you weigh less than 150 pounds, 35 pounds if your weight is 150-200 pounds, and 45 pounds if you weigh more than 200. Adding weight beyond that is not going to make the exercise any more productive. As long as the counterweight has "taken your legs from underneath you", you are set.

The required weight will also be affected by your bodyweight distribution. The more top heavy you are, the fewer plates you will need, and vice versa. So don't be surprised when ladies use more weight. (Another reason not to compare your Hardstyle sit-up performance with someone else's—your wife or girlfriend will trash you.)

The above numbers are guidelines, not hard rules. Your goal is to eventually find the weight that gives you the most intense abdominal contraction.

The Ab Pavelizer™ is not your typical pretty boy ab machine. Even the first version of the device stopped one of the most famous powerlifters in the world cold at just three reps and most experienced bodybuilders could not do a single one. Measurements from Prof. McGill's lab show that the Ab Pavelizer™ gets an extraordinary rectus abdominis contraction exceeding 175% MVC (maximal voluntary isometric contraction)! In other words, if you purposefully tense your abs as hard as possible, the Ab Pavelizer™ will make them tense almost twice as hard!

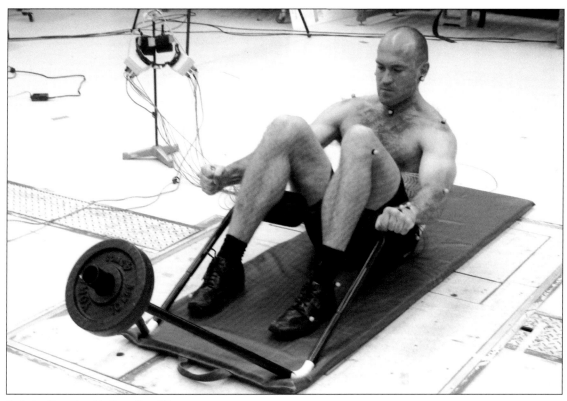

Lab testing the Ab Pavelizer™
Courtesy Prof. Stuart McGill's Spine Biomechanics Lab at the University of Waterloo, Canada

Following are some readings we recorded. Here is my EMG, with the darkest line indicating the activity of the "six-pack":

Pavelizer Sit-up—Tense Glutes Bring Tail Bone and Sacrum Together (45lb)

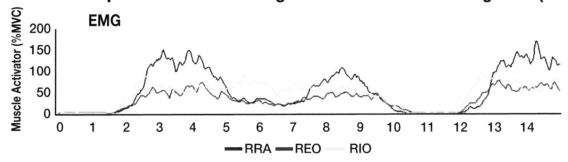

That is some serious recruitment and tension, which directly translate into full body strength and an armored six-pack. Renowned strength coach Mike Burgener, former elite weightlifter and father and coach of elite weightlifters, states: "The Ab Pavelizer is the only device that I use with my athletes to build strong functional abdominals. My athletes range from 16 year-old weightlifters to 74 year-old geezers. We use the Ab Pavelizer in all our workouts. We train abs three times per week and normally hit 3-4 sets of 5-10 reps. I cannot believe the strength we gain in our abs using the Ab Pavelizer... it IS ABSOLUTELY THE BEST AB STRENGTHENER I HAVE FOUND!!! Just hard ass work that really develops the core!!!" Mike is very old school and not prone to exaggeration.

If a Partner or Equipment are not an Option: for Advanced Hardstylers Only

If even a rubber band is not around, do your Hardstyle sit-ups without any equipment. It is below sauerkraut on the food chain—down there with chicken?—but it is better than not doing this powerful exercise at all. When no one and nothing is pulling on your calves you have to really watch out that your lower back does not arch and your abs and glutes are tensed! Specialists warn: "The arching of the back stretches the abdominal muscles, and they may appear firm under tension. The examiner must be careful not to mistake this tautness for firmness due to actual contraction of the muscles."[39] Which is why I do not recommend it to anyone who does not already have the Hardstyle sit-up down pat and abs to kill for. If Ab Pavelizer™ is not an option, hook a rubber band to the doorknob and feed it around your calves. There is a saying in Russia: "Sauerkraut is good to serve with vodka. It is not embarrassing to put on the table, yet it is cheap and you throw away the leftovers with an easy heart." (It sounds better in Russian.) A rubber band is "sauerkraut". Experienced gymnast Moses Dungca comments that a rubber band "is just 'similar' and not the same thing as the Pavelizer. Again, the PAVELIZER is the finest device I've have ever come across. It is what it is and there is really nothing else like it.

Moses adds another reason the Ab Pavelizer™ rules (the italics are mine): "I fully recommend the Ab Pavelizer... It's the 'real deal' and there is nothing like it. It's evil and it's supposed to be that way. Trust me, *you'll understand how to truly use and activate your abdominals* once you try it. There is nothing like it. AND... I was a gymnast. My abdominals never felt that way before."

What Dungca refers to is the "reverse engineering of strength" for which my system is known. "Hardstyle", which is an umbrella term for all my teachings (kettlebell, barbell, bodyweight, mobility, flexibility, etc.), views strength as a skill and **reverse engineers the body language of the strongest people in the world.** (Thanks to Louie Simmons of the Westside Barbell Club, I can finally explain what I do in one sentence.)

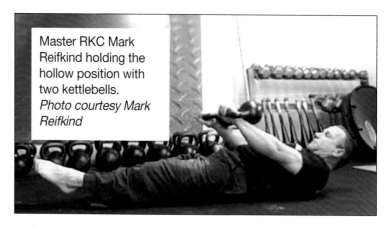

Master RKC Mark Reifkind holding the hollow position with two kettlebells. *Photo courtesy Mark Reifkind*

The Hardstyle sit-up reverse engineers a key element of the body language of the athlete with the most spectacular set of abs—the gymnast. Watch him perform an elite ring exercise like the iron cross. You can't help noticing a Pavelizer like contraction of the abs and glutes.

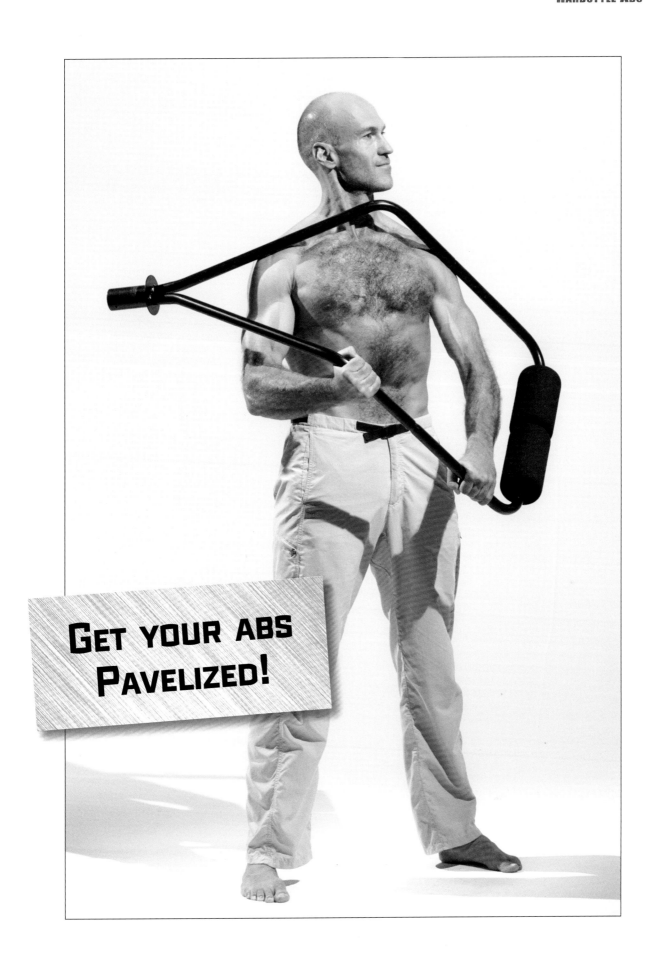

GET YOUR ABS
PAVELIZED!

FOOTNOTES

19 Kendall et al. (1971)

20 Juker et al. (1998)

21 Kendall et al. (2005)

22 Bret Contreras comments: "A glute contraction protects against shear through tension of the thoracolumbar fascia, which has excellent leverage for anti-flexion (Sullivan, 1989). It is my belief that this is a huge reason why powerlifters could round back deadlift without blowing out discs; their strong glutes contract hard, which tenses the TLF, which counteracts a significant portion of the flexion moment. (Vleeming et al., 1995)"

23 O'Sullivan et al. (1997)

24 Tesh et al. (1987), McGill (1998), McGill (2001)

25 Semyonov (1968)

26 While breath holding is enough to work the obliques, it takes sharp cough like exhalations to get the six-pack's attention. From Basmajian & DeLuca (1985): "When the subjects… were made to strain or to bear down" with the breath held, the external obliques and the internal obliques (lower parts) contracted to a degree that was directly related to the effort, but rectus abdominis, in contrast, was very quiet. (Floyd & Silver, 1950) This was later confirmed by Ono (1958)… de Sousa & Furlani (1974)… found exuberant activity by the recti bilaterally during a cough. So there is a difference, apparently, between the reactions of the recti to the increase of intra-abdominal pressure from "bearing down" and sharp, short increase of coughing."

27 McGill (2009)

28 Zakharyants (1962)

29 Verkhoshansky & Siff (2009)

30 Herrington (2011). The data is for the "normal asymptomatic population".

31 Herrington (2011)

32 Prof. Stuart McGill was kind enough to add his commentary:

> Here is a summary of spine motion or non-neutral postures. If the spine is under load, the discs will succumb faster if they are bent (non-neutral postures). If the load is lower this is not much of a concern. So any "pulsing" of muscle activity will be better tolerated when the spine is closer to neutral. Having stated that, motion while loaded is more risky than locking the spine in a non-neutral posture when under load. Consider picking up an Atlas stone from the ground —deep squat and full spine flexion—but the torso is wrapped around the stone in a flexed but isometric grip on the stone. This is less risky than moving the spine under such a great load.

> I also make the distinction between those that have back injury and those who have never had an injury—many do not get this distinction but you certainly do. If there is an injury history it must be managed and a lot of our strategies are to manage the injury and remain functional. So I will be insistent for the flexion intolerant back that they have to avoid this at all costs— yet for others it is not so important. As always— these are individual considerations.

> Also, the tolerable volume of training is modulated by the spine posture. Repeated bending of the spine reduces the tolerable volume—for example one could tolerate much more volume in "stir the pot" on a ball vs situps. But as you point out the idea is to train less for better athleticism—your synopsis on this is about the best I have read—very well done!

33 While Russian researchers do not question the fact that isometrics build strength (Vorobyev, 1977), they consider it only a supplementary strength training modality (Zatsiorsky, 1996). Isometrics should constitute only 10% of the strength training volume (Vorobyev & Slobodyan, 1977). A mix of muscle work regimes needs to be employed in order to continue improving results (Semyonov & Chudinov, 1963; Petrov & Chudinov, 1966).

34 Shields & Heiss (1997), Drysdale et al. (2004), Urquhart et al. (2005)

35 Workman et al. (2008)

36 McGill (2006)

37 Sarti et al. (1996), Willet et al. (2001)

38 Lipetz & Gutin (1970), Guimaraes et al. (1991)

39 Kendall et al. (1971)

Internal Isometrics:
the secret of old time physical culturalists' exceptional abdominal strength and development

> ### THE THOUGHTS ARE THE STRENGTH
> ### OF MY MUSCLES.
> ### —PRENTICE MULFORD

Once you can do 5x5 full range Hardstyle sit-ups, how do you progress?

Certainly not by adding reps and not by adding weight either. The answer is trying to tense your muscles harder. Several years ago Steve Maxwell suggested to the trainees doing modified Janda situps: "Don't see how many reps you can do, see how *few* you can do!" Indeed, the higher is the tension, the quicker the onset of fatigue. So the stronger you get, the quicker you get gassed. After just one or two I am toast. Whatever reps you manage, if you feel that the tension is about to drop off—you are done. This is the mindset of strength—the opposite of the mindset of endurance—to give it all at once.

This is a good time to stress that the Hardstyle sit-up is an exercise and not a lift and you should not compare your numbers to someone else's—or even to your own for that matter! Find some other way of evaluating your abdominal strength progress if you must—say, the L-seat on parallel bars for time or the number of consecutive hollow rocks—but don't chase any sort of numerical improvement in your Hardstyle sit-up.

Back to progression. There are several reasons why I don't like adding weight to forward flexion exercises. In the case of Hardstyle sit-ups, physics will not allow you to add much—you would just tip over. And in the case of Swiss ball crunches, regular sit-ups, and the like, I don't care for the logistical challenge. Paul Chek has used over 200 pounds in the former. A manly effort in an effective exercise. If you are willing to put up with the hassle and have a reliable ball and spotter—power to you. I will pass, I am lazy, I am Russian.

Powerlifter Bruce Anderson decided to get serious about his abs. He started doing straight-legged sit-ups with a 25-pound plate. Five years later he was up to 435 pounds of plates for a set of 10! Another effort worthy of admiration but I am not so sure about emulation. Again, I have nothing against the exercise or its effectiveness, I am just dreading dealing with all these wheels.

I would make an exception for the hanging leg raise—snapping on a couple of ankle weights is not as bothersome as piling hundreds of pounds on your chest—but since most athletes cannot even do a single rep of the proper HLR unweighted, this is mostly theoretical. Besides, even studs can find plenty of challenging HLR variations without adding weight.

It is not that I don't believe in adding weight—I just think it is not worth it. Save those wheels for your deadlifts. And in the case of less than elite athletes loading up is pointless: adding weight to crunches made no difference in ab recruitment in female college students.[40]

So if we don't add reps or weight, what is the alternative?—Increasing the intensity of contraction.

Scientists differentiate between *external isometrics* and *internal isometrics*. "The former refers to isometric contraction exerted against an external load, whereas the latter refers to contraction exerted against opposing muscles within the body, much like muscle posing actions performed by bodybuilders."[41] In my opinion, the impressive abs you see on the top guys are not the result of their high rep crunches but of their posing. They also know how to develop a "mind to muscle link" and really focus on squeezing those abbies. As should you.

Prof. McGill, when teaching his patented "McGill curl-up" to elite athletes, instructs: "Even the most serious athletes can increase the challenge… to ultimate training levels. First, a pre-brace is performed by the entire abdominal wall. It is maximally activated—neither sucked in nor blown out. The secret is to curl… against the abdominal brace in such a way that the large resistance is provided by the activated abdominals…"

In addition to the obvious resistance of the "bubble" of intra-abdominal pressure created by Hardstyle breathing[42]—you are fighting your own lower back muscles. It is fascinating that increasing the IAP reflexively makes the spinal erectors contract "vigorously", even in full flexion.[43] At McGill's lab my lower erectors reached 80% peak activation during a variation of the Hardstyle breathing drill practiced by Russian boxers—while they barely passed 55% when I was deadlifting 80% of the max I was capable of at that time! No wonder Hardstyle sit-ups are so hard—you are fighting the resistance of your very strong lower back muscles. Who needs extra weight?

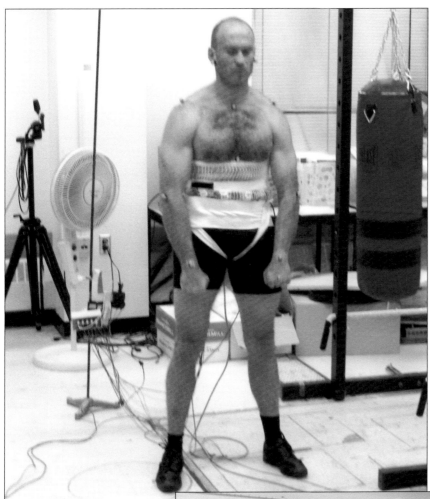

A Hardstyle breathing drill made the lower back muscles contract a lot harder than a 405-pound beltless deadlift! *Courtesy Prof. Stuart McGill's Spine Biomechanics Lab at the University of Waterloo, Canada*

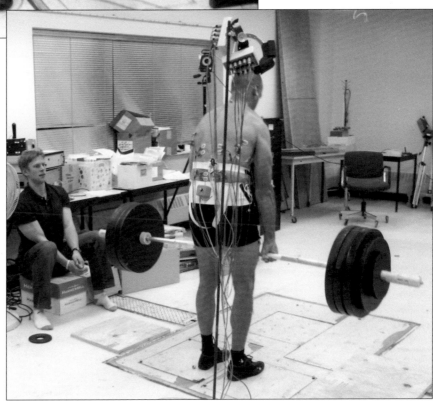

In addition to straining against the brace and the bubble simply try to maximally tense all of the muscles of the abdominal wall. A variation of internal isometrics is the unfortunately forgotten "muscle control" method, which requires one to maximally contract individual muscles using nothing but will power. One of its most famous practitioners, European strongman and physique man Maxick, recalled his amazing transformation:

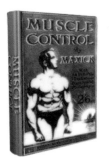

In my daily association with my schoolmates I was always the weakest in our play activities. My natural boy's feelings rebelled against the superiority of the others and the desire grew in me to become far stronger than they... I with the assistance of several friends managed to make a stone dumbbell. This crude dumbbell, however, had only a short span of life. My father, who neither knew nor approved of my secret plans, smashed it into a thousand pieces. However, I was far from allowing myself to be discouraged by this and other setbacks in the future. At night, when all other members of my family abandoned themselves to refreshing sleep, I remained awake in my bed and tried to replace the demolished dumbbell by tensing and relaxing different muscle groups.

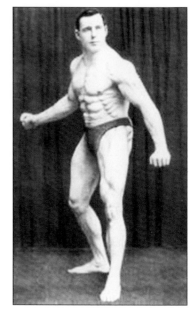

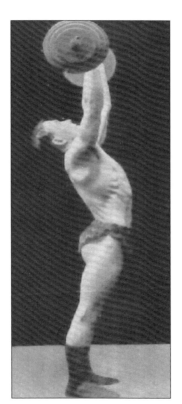

I very soon learned that the important factor was the inspiration of determination in performing an exercise and not merely the number of repetitions. With this I want to say that I did not put any special value on a high number of mechanical repetitions but that I combined every individual movement with the conscious sensing of a strengthening of a certain group of muscles. Through this process the entire attention flowed into the muscles active at the moment and the inner expectation of a strengthening resulted in an advantageous change of the physique.

It is known that everything men have created has first been shaped and imagined in the idea and in thoughts. The strength, however, which is necessary for the materialization of a thought is the intensity with which we inspire that thought and with which we finally mold it into a form perceptible to the senses.

Dan Cenidoza, RKC who implemented muscle control into his training regimen several years ago with great success, muses, "I am no longer sure about the cliché, "Your body knows movements not muscles." I see no reason that you cannot know both. I understand why people say that, to encourage new trainees to think of exercise in terms of movements instead of bodypart muscle building, but if movements are a skill, that makes both muscular contractions and the neural counterpart that drives it a skill as well." Well said, Comrade.

This focus on the muscles works. Fellow strongman Tromp Van Diggelen had more than a few words to say about Maxick and his ability:

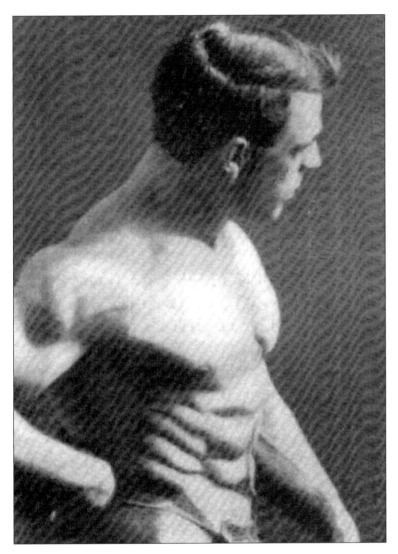

No photograph can do him justice, he has a "quality" of muscle which is absolutely unique. When contracting his muscles, he looks like an anatomical chart, yet when I used to massage him... his muscles felt like soft wet chamois leather in my hands.

*...Max, who usually weighed **under** 140 pounds in his music-hall performances, would invite any heavy man in the audience who would like to be lifted to come on the stage. This human dynamo would even take a 240 pound man, apply his open palm to the man's lower spine, get the man to grip his (Max's) wrist with both hands, then he would hoist the cumbersome human dumbbell to his shoulder using his left hand to help and then without any fuss push him to arm's length (using the one arm only) and walk off the stage with him.*

Here is another feat of speed and almost atomic energy which [Maxick] accomplished laughingly: He would take an empty champagne bottle, fill it three quarters full of water, grip it tightly by the neck with his left hand and then give the open mouth a smart tap with his right palm; he never failed to knock the bottom out, except when the bottle just collapsed in a general way. Just get a hold of a champagne bottle and try this feat, it will give you some idea of the unusual dynamic strength my buddy had...

...Max side pressed me (185 pounds) above his head supporting me (on my back) on his open palm, no less than 16 times; in his left hand he held a glass of beer filled to the brim with his arm stretched at right angles to his body and he did not spill a drop!... Here is just another "stunt" that even Saxon would have found hard, I used to lie with my back on Max's open palm and he would tell me to close my eyes and it is honestly true that I would not know I was at arm's length until he told me to open my eyes.

To show the terrific strength of his abdominal muscles Sick used to lie flat on stage and I, or some other 180 or 200 pound man, would stand 7 feet above him and jump on his abdomen; believe me, I bounced as if jumping on to solid rubber! You mathematicians can work out with what force the feet of a 200 pound man would strike Max's rectus abdominis when falling from a height of 7 feet.[44]

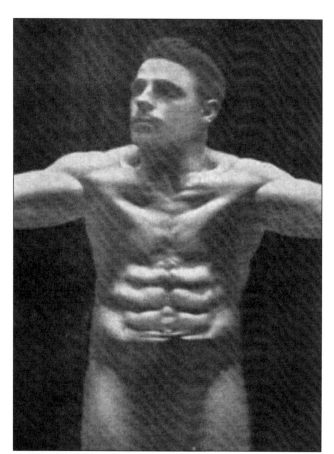

[Maxick] 'commanded' (that is the word for it) each muscle of his body. His will seemed to act as commander-in-chief... A famous anatomist once said to me: "When Sick does feats of strength he actually seems to exceed his physical powers" and it is true that his mental concentration is something phenomenal... the 'quality' of his muscle is such as I have never seen before or since and I have examined many hundreds of real strong men."

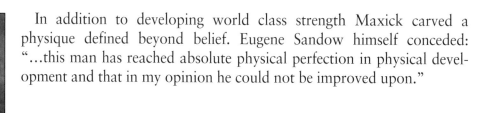

Eugene Sandow

In addition to developing world class strength Maxick carved a physique defined beyond belief. Eugene Sandow himself conceded: "...this man has reached absolute physical perfection in physical development and that in my opinion he could not be improved upon."

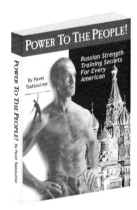

I hope you are convinced that directing your attention to squeezing your abs harder will make you strong and look the part. Here is an additional benefit to consider. I have explained the benefits of *feed-forward tension*—the skill of getting super tight before one's body is loaded—in ***Power to the People!*** and ***The Naked Warrior***. Powerlifters, arm-wrestlers, and gymnasts are masters of feed-forward tension because isometrically pre-tensing the muscles before a dynamic contraction can improve one's performance by up to 20%![45]

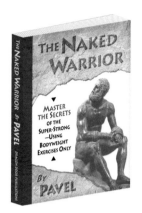

Rif explains:

This is feed-forward tension, the real domain of the gymnast. What makes gymnasts look like they are moving so effortlessly is the fact that they can get tight and stay tight as long as they need to. When you see "form" breaks on a gymnast, what you are see-

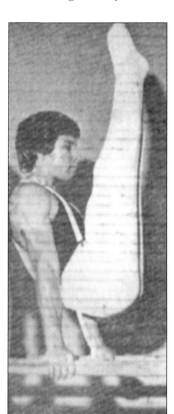

ing is the lack of the athlete in keeping his body tight. In order to do these incredibly complicated movements (or even simple ones like handstands) the body has to be made into as few "segments" as necessary to complete the task. When one is flipping through the air the fewer "pieces" the body is broken into, the easier it is to more move around. Think of a shovel that has a bend in the middle of it. Not much use as a lever, is it? Same for a gymnast who gets soft in the core, or the glutes, or anywhere... The next time you see a gymnast on the rings doing ANYTHING, much less an advanced strength skill such as an Iron Cross, a front or back lever you will have a much greater respect for the "unseen" strength of these incredible athletes.

Developing the skill of greatly tensing the midsection and the glutes without external resistance is an important aspect of reverse engineering a gymnast's strength and physique. Don't bother adding weight or reps. Just add tension.

Master RKC Mark Reifkind was one of the top gymnasts in the USA in the 1970s, going head to head with Kurt Thomas.
Courtesy Mark Reifkind

FOOTNOTES

40 Morales et al. (2003)

41 Verkhoshansky & Siff (2009)

42 "Intra-abdominal pressure produces spinal extension…" (Zatsiorsky, 1995)

43 Floyd & Silver (1955). Basmaijan & De Luca (1985) comment: "The clinical implications of this last observation have not been, from our point of view, adequately explored by orthopedic specialists." To me this explains why a gymnast who has never touched a barbell is usually able to deadlift an impressive poundage the first time out. Food for thought for the bodyweight only types: high tension abdominal and full body exercises will probably strengthen your lower back more than back extensions, bridges, and the like.

44 Bret Contreras: "Okay I'll bite—I'm a math geek. A 90kg (198lb) man falling 7ft (2.13m) will have a velocity of 6.5m/s (14.5 mph) and a kinetic energy of 1,879J right before impact. If this impact is absorbed over a .0508m (2 inch) deformation of the abdominals, this equates to 36,981N (8,314 pounds) of force."

45 Verkhoshansky & Siff (2009)

The Hardstyle Hanging Leg Raise:
no sissies need apply

have never known a single person who regularly practiced hanging leg raises and failed to develop a hard and useful set of abs. Ever. The HLR belongs in the training schedule of any hard Comrade.

HLRs are the cornerstone of gymnasts' abdominal training—so they obviously have a proven track record of producing world-class abs.

Because of its difficulty and effectiveness the HLR was the midsection drill of choice in the underground gyms of Lyubertsi in the 1980s. Street toughs from this small town in the greater Moscow were feared for their rare combo of fighting skills and muscle.

Russian powerlifters and power bodybuilders are convinced that this drill is a fine addition to a powerlifter's regimen. Squat world record holder in the 181-pound class Igor Shestakov starts and finishes his workouts with 2x20 strict HLRs and has an extraordinarily developed midsection as a bonus to go with his world record.

Elite bodybuilders got on the bar as well. The HLR is the favorite abdominal move of Mr. Olympia Jay Cutler: "Hanging leg raises are the key to midsection development, and are obviously the hardest to do, especially when your legs weigh 200 pounds." (They don't and make up about 1/3 of one's bodyweight, but the poor leverage imposed by their length makes them feel like they do.)

The HLR works the waist super-intensely with peak activation reaching 163% for the EO and 300% for the lower RA![46]

There are a dozen other great reasons to pursue HLRs I can think of. I will hit them one at a time, when you are resting between your sets.

Let us establish what constitutes a legit HLR:

- The arms remain straight at all times
- Look straight ahead and do not tilt your head back
- Start from a dead hang and move at a controlled, momentum free cadence
- Keep the legs straight or nearly straight
- Touch your shins or feet to the bar

Anything less is wishful thinking.

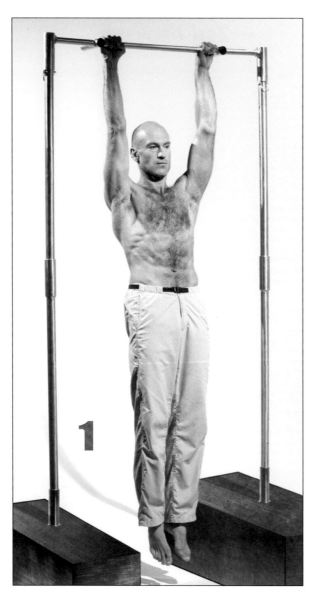

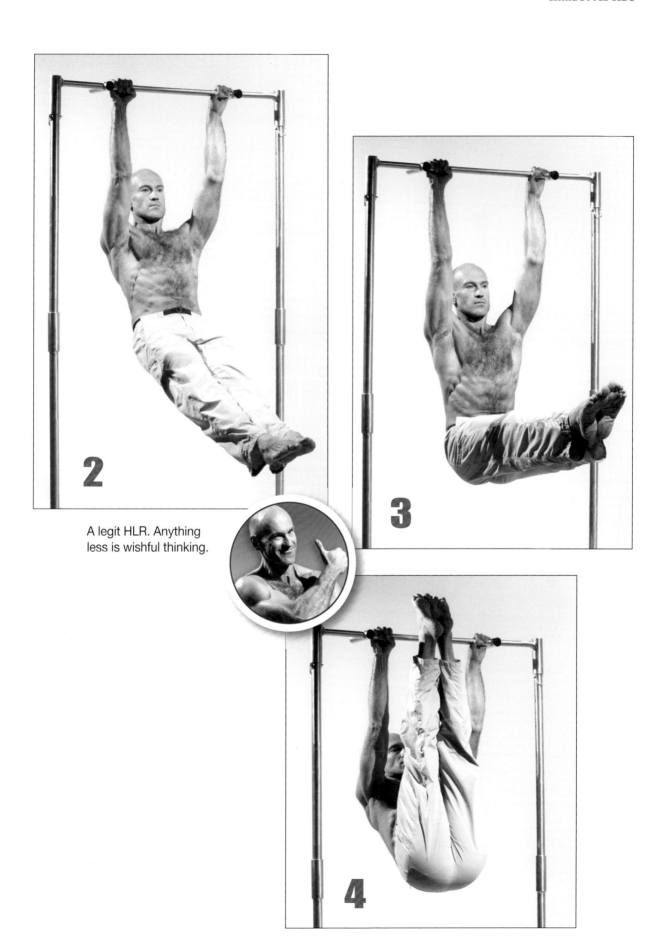

2

A legit HLR. Anything less is wishful thinking.

3

4

Needless to say, you will not be starting there. Months of Hardstyle breathing and Hardstyle sit-ups must come first. As well as flexibility training for your hamstrings and, to a lesser degree, for your back. If you can't touch your toes while keeping your legs straight standing or sitting on the ground, you will not stand a chance up on the bar. Don't undertake HLRs until your toe touches are adequate.

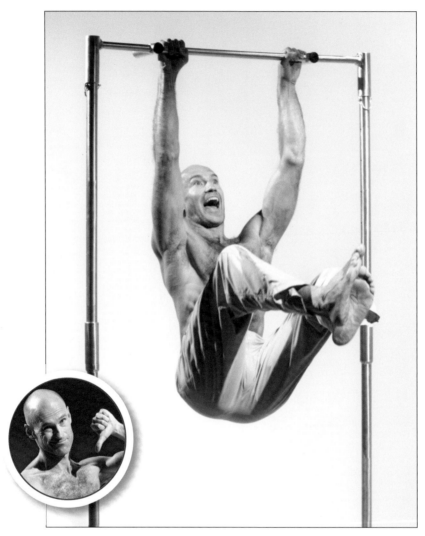

You have got to be kidding me, Comrade!

The next step is learning to take the arch out of your lower back and the slack out of your body to assume the so-called "hollow position" from gymnastics. British gymnastics coach Lloyd Readhead stresses that this position is "essential to the safe and successful development of a great number of gymnastic skills and the ability to retain this shape must be developed throughout the gymnast's career."

I will remind you that "hollow" does not refer to sucking in your stomach! This posture looks like a very open "C": the athlete's straight arms and legs are stretched out like a diver's but the tension in his abs "shrinks" the front of the body and brings the arms and the legs towards each other a little. The tailbone is maximally tucked in and the chest is sunk in. Not a pretty posture but a strong one.[47]

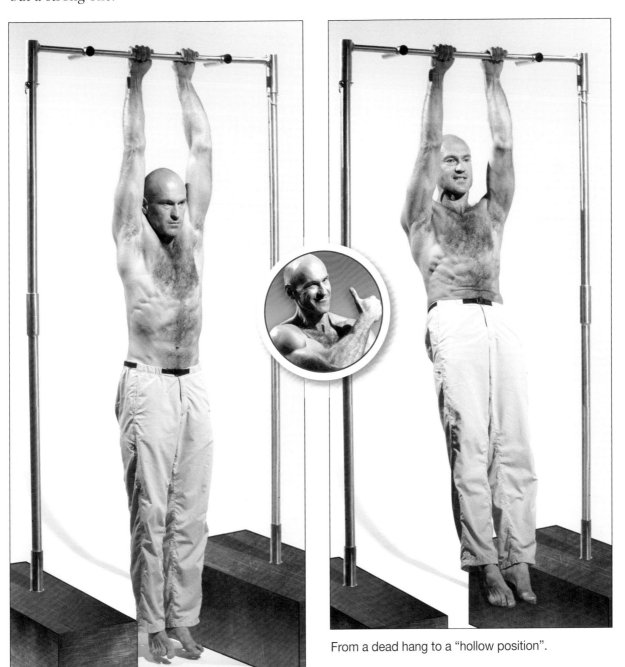

From a dead hang to a "hollow position".

We have a special way of learning the hollow position: hang on a pullup bar and Hardstyle breathe. Use a narrow grip: you should be able to almost touch the tips of your thumbs together if you tried. Comrades with huge upper bodies will have to go wider, but they still should grip narrower than their shoulders. The purpose of this narrow grip is to pre-stretch your lats and thus unload your shoulders. Another Hardstyle subtlety to fire up your lats even more, is to use a thumbless grip.

It is even better to start this and all other HLR progressions on narrow, shoulder width or slightly narrower, parallel bars. The semi-supinated grip makes the exercise easier and is friendlier to the shoulders. Not a bad choice when you are learning the moves.

Your arms must be straight at all times in this drill and in all other HLR evolutions. Flexing the elbows reduces the effectiveness of the exercise and threatens the shoulders. A Hardstyle tip: tense your triceps and keep them tensed.

Keep your legs straight as well, your kneecaps pulled up and your toes pointed. For greater effectiveness squeeze a small water bottle, empty but with a cap on, between your legs: right above or below the knees or between the ankles. This dramatically increases the midsection tension. Feel free to use the water bottle in your hanging leg raises as well, when you get there. It also works like a charm for pullups. Instructors at one of the federal law enforcement agencies that hire me as a subject matter expert have had great success boosting their recruits' pullups with this simple technique.

Take a breath and start Hardstyle breathing in the familiar manner of ramping up short hisses. It will be a lot harder than on the ground, as now your midsection muscles, in addition to their usual challenges, have to fight the gravity to bring your pelvis closer to your ribcage. Try to shorten that distance by contracting your abs and your external obliques. If you have done everything correctly, at the end of the Hardstyle exhalation the bottom of the ribcage ought to flatten out to form a straight line with the stomach—no more, no less.

Don't forget the familiar elements of Hardstyle breathing: tucking in your tail, performing the karate navel maneuver, etc.

Your body will "shrink". Your legs will naturally come up a little as a result of this shortening of the muscles on the front of your torso: the "dish" shape of the hollow position. Let them but don't make them; you do not want to use your hip flexors just yet.

Jump off, rest for a minute or so, then do another rep with new elements added: the action of your shoulders and lats.

One of the great benefits of the HLR is that it integrates the lats and other muscles involved in extending the shoulders (pushing the arms down) with the midsection muscles. Without going into details, your lats are a part of your "core" and stabilizing the spine is one of their responsibilities. Even if you are a pretty boy with no interest in performance, contracting the lats makes your abs tense harder. Exercises in which the arms are fixed and the shoulder extensors are activated—like the HLR—"facilitate activation of the abdominal musculature".[48] Indeed, the straight-arm pull-down—one hardly thinks of it as an abdominal move—beat the crunch by 14% when it came to the rectus abdominis contraction.[49] (This should give you a hint why pullups are such a powerful ab developer.)

There are several steps in reverse engineering an elite gymnast's coordination of the lats, serratus anterior, subscapularis, and other muscles responsible for pushing down on the bar. Have patience, it is worth it. Add one step at a time.

The first step is "packing your shoulders"—a pure safety measure. Just pull your arms into the shoulder sockets—but don't pull your shoulder blades down. (For the nerds amongst you: depress the glenohumeral joints, not the scapulae. Don't retract the scapulae either.)

The second step is pushing your straight arms down, as if you are trying to do a straight-arm pull-down or a front lever. This will engage many muscles on the front of your torso and in your armpits. If your abbies are strong and your movement patterns are normal, this will reflexively amplify the intensity of the abdominal contraction.[50]

Do not be tempted to look up at this or any other point of the hanging leg raise—look straight ahead. Don't extend your neck either.

These Hardstyle subtleties may take you awhile to master but they will pay off big.

The third step is attempting to "break the bar", as taught in *The Naked Warrior*, to get some external shoulder rotation and to fire up the lats and other "armpit muscles". Another cue meant to accomplish the same goal is trying to "make the elbows face each other". Of course, unless you have been worked over by a BJJ champion, it is not possible. But the intention will recruit the right muscles. Do not let your hands move or elbows flex when you are "breaking the bar" or "making the elbows face each other".

The fourth action is squeezing your arms together to activate the pecs as if you are crushing an old-fashioned Bullworker device. Masterfully engaging the chest in "pulling" exercises is one of the secrets of gymnasts' awesome upper body strength. If you take a few minutes to ponder the direction in which the pec major pulls, it should no longer surprise you.

Perform all of these actions as you are Hardstyle breathing and tensing your abs, your glutes, your legs. If you do everything by the book, by the end each rep your body will feel like a solid block of wood, every muscle from your toes to your hands linked in an unbreakable chain. This is Hardstyle.

Practice hanging Hardstyle breathing for 5-10 sets with plenty of rest in between. After a few lessons, when you feel that you have it down pat, add a partial leg raise to it.

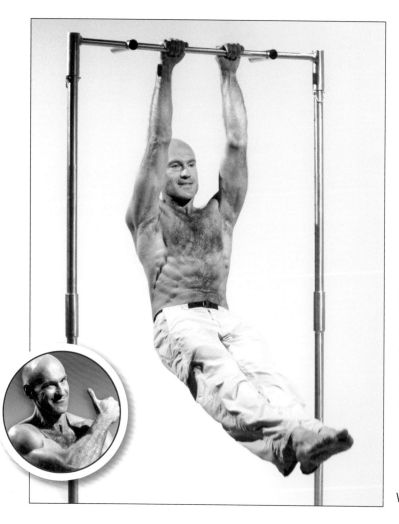

Hiss out only once or twice and start raising your legs slowly while maintaining the abdominal brace you have just achieved. Let the breathing take care of itself at this point. Hardstyle breathing throughout the whole rep of an HLR will have to wait until you get a lot stronger. Pressurizing your abdomen makes every strength exercise easier—except spinal flexion ones. Recall that increased IAP produces spine extension via two mechanisms: pneumatic-hydraulic and reflexive activation of the back extensors. Therefore Hardstyle breathing will make the HLR much harder and it already is hard enough. Hence after a short hiss or two to take the slack out of the body, breathe or do not breathe as feels natural.

When ready, add a partial leg raise.

It is imperative that you do not let your lower back arch as you raise your legs! If it does, you have not earned the right to do leg raises. Your abs and especially external obliques must be strong and smart enough to counter the pull of the powerful hip flexors.

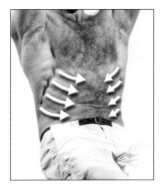

Ponder the direction of contraction of the external obliques.

The obliques have the reputation for twisting the trunk or bending it sideways. They do all that but if the EO on both sides contract at the same time they give the RA and the glutes a hand in tilting your pelvis posteriorly. Imagine sliding both hands into the pockets of a tight fitting leather jacket. The hands are the EO. Imagine how they shorten and tilt the front of the pelvis towards your head. Interestingly, even if you are strong at sit-ups, leg raises might be out of your league, and not just because of the poor leverage imposed by these long limbs, but because of the extra demands on the external obliques imposed by the body's complex engineering.[51] Ironically, too many sit-ups might make you weaker at leg raises![52] To add to the challenge, unlike in the Hardstyle sit-up, the glutes are not in position to help the EO and RA as much in tucking in the tail to prevent spine extension.

Raise your legs as high as you can without resorting to back arching, momentum, or leaning back. Just a few inches are good enough for now. At this stage of the game your best bet is to do single repetitions. Better get a tighter contraction and a higher leg raise than more reps.

Master RKC Jeff O'Connor offers tips on mastering this phase of the hanging leg raise: "The key here is to "let go" of the glutes at just the right time. Focus on cramping the glutes until the legs rise as high as possible, then shift your focus to pulling up the kneecaps.... Work on this until you can make a seamless transition... The final step is to add max tension from the top. As the legs rise, visualize pulling the bar to the feet."

You must understand that you will not get very far if you simply try to raise your legs. The HLR action is a jackknife. In other words, as you are lifting your legs you should be "lowering'" your shoulders by pressing down on the bar with your arms. This demand is what makes the HLR so effective at "knitting together" into a big pullup.

So keep pushing down on the bar as you are bringing your legs up. Keep your knees locked or almost locked. Flexing them makes the exercise a lot easier and less effective. Did I say stretch your hamstrings? It would not hurt to do it right before your HLR sessions. As a side note, the HLR is an assessment of one's body composition and active flexibility. One needs a dangerous blend of strength and flexibility and no gut in order to achieve it.

What to Do When no Pullup Bar is Around

A gymnast's favorite, "hollow rocks".

Assume the hollow position on the floor. Straighten your legs, tense them, and squeeze them together. Point your toes. Have your pelvis, lower back, abs and glutes do what they do in the Hardstyle sit-up: tuck and cramp. Lift your sunk in chest and your head slightly off the ground. Try to limit the upper back and neck movement—remember the relevant instructions for the Hardstyle sit-up.

Press your tongue into the roof of your mouth behind the front teeth to reflexively activate the proper neck stabilizing pattern.[53]

Several arms positions are possible. The easiest is to have your hands on your chest or "on guard". The standard version is with your arms stretched along your body, as if ready to grab a bar. Better yet, hold a broomstick, as suggested by Will Williams. You may also employ McGill's "superstiffness" technique: press your palms, both facing the ceiling, against each other.

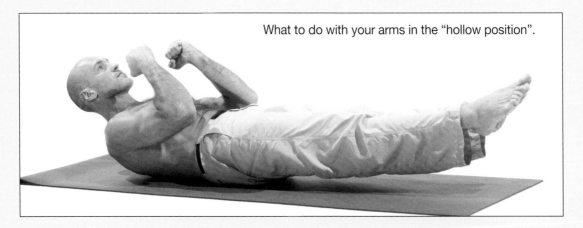

What to do with your arms in the "hollow position".

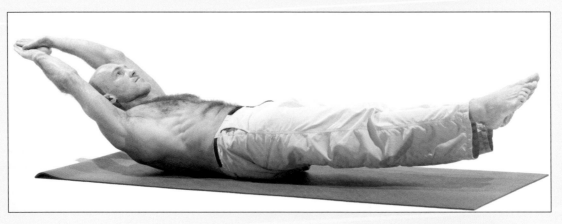

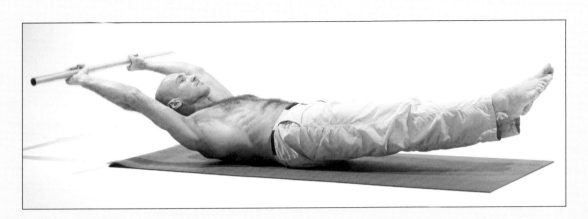

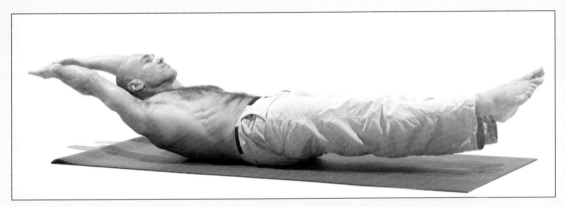

Breathe shallow and rock back and forth without losing this position. Your body must remain one stiff piece—there should be no movement in the hips, ribs, or lower back whatsoever, no stretching of the abs. Movement indicates weakness. Unlike in the hanging leg raises and Hardstyle sit-ups where the abs are prime or assistant movers, in hollow rocks they are stabilizers. And, as Gray Cook has put it in his classic book *Movement*, "Stabilizers'… role is *not to move* in the presence of movement…"

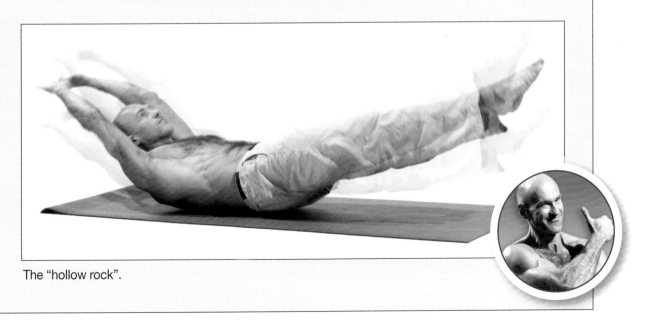

The "hollow rock".

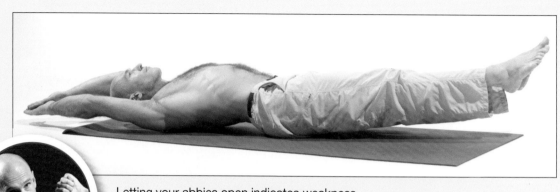

Letting your abbies open indicates weakness.

Rif recommends multiple sets of 10-15sec with the same amount of rest between sets. "Serious work here," he promises.

Rolling side to side, from cheek to cheek, is another variation of the hollow drill. Make sure your upper and lower body roll as a unit, with no delay.

Whether you are hollow "rocking" or "rolling", you may squeeze a water bottle, empty or filled, with a cap on between your ankles.

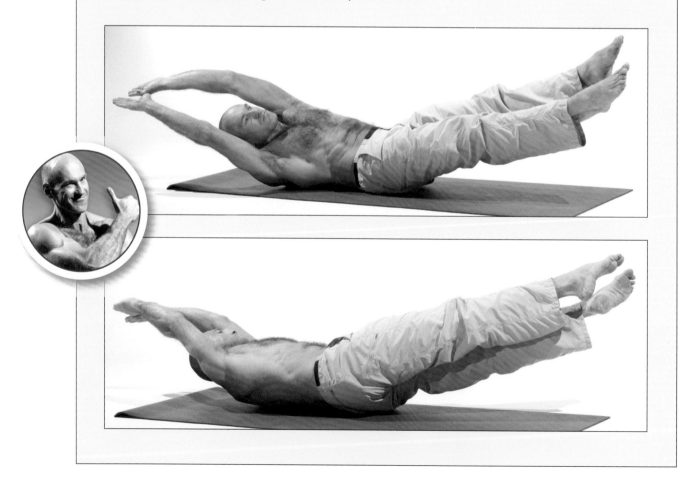

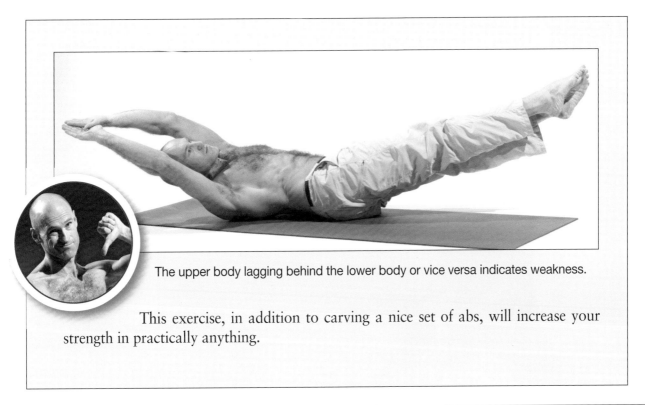

The upper body lagging behind the lower body or vice versa indicates weakness.

This exercise, in addition to carving a nice set of abs, will increase your strength in practically anything.

Just as practicing partial pullups is not likely to enable you to do a full one, partial HLRs will help but will not take you all the way. Hanging knee raises, although they seem like a natural regression, are a waste of time. The feeling of this exercise is too different from the real deal HLR. Russian and Bulgarian gymnastics coaches solve the problem with a contraption similar to the Total Gym®. Chuck Norris should not feel embarrassed to endorse this product. Many Russian gymnasiums are equipped with stall bars, wooden ladder like contraptions mounted on the wall. This old-fashioned rig is very versatile for strength and flexibility training. Relevant to our cause, it usually comes with a six-foot long board with hooks on one end. You park one end of the board on the floor and hook the top on a stall bar at your chosen level. A cart, big enough to park your upper body on comfort-

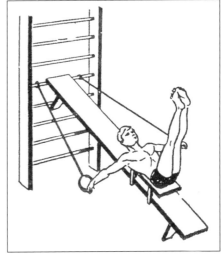

ably, slides up and down the board on wheels. This contraption enables even the weakest to perform hard moves like the handstand pushup and even the iron cross. Adjust the angle of the board to your strength level—the flatter the board, the easier the exercise—and you are in business. The coach will mount a set of gymnastic rings near the athlete's head, and the latter will be able to do a perfect cross! Soviet research is definite: this approach of performing the target exercise in a properly unloaded manner is far superior to the traditional method of simultaneous general strength training and lead-up exercises.[54]

The hanging leg raise is built in the same manner: start with the board flat on the floor, hold onto the bar, and go. As you get stronger, progressively elevate the head. This works great, the only problem is: stall bars, not to mention boards with carts, are not to be found in the US. So I was guilty of pushing ineffective hanging knee raises on unsuspecting Americans until I finally figured out a way to use standard US gym equipment. A power rack—or even a training partner and a broomstick—is all you need.

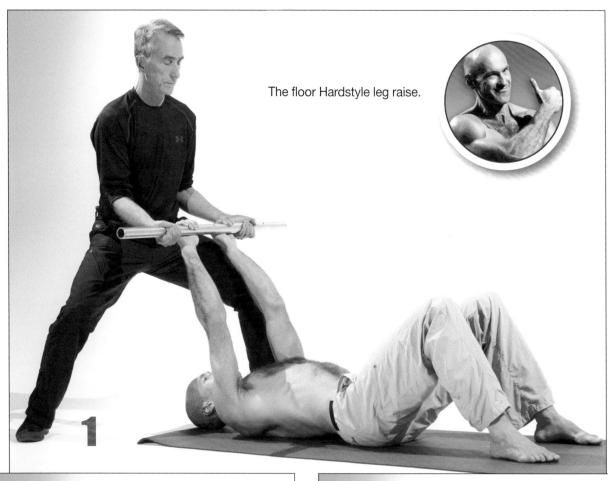

The floor Hardstyle leg raise.

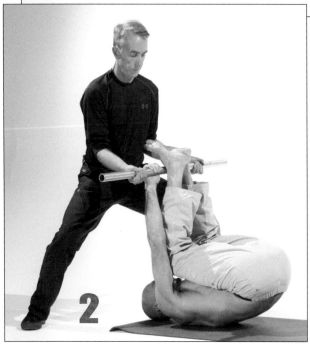

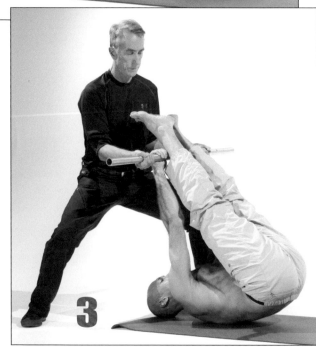

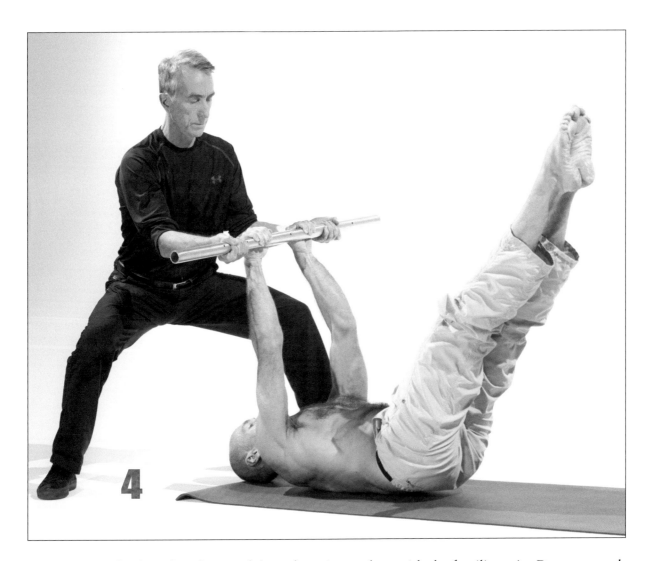

Lie on your back and grab one of the safety pins set low with the familiar grip. Do not stretch your arms in line with the body like a diver. Gymnasts refer to the above position as the "open shoulders". While this is your eventual goal, today you will train with relatively "closed shoulders" (less flexion), with your elbows approximately at your eye level. This is a much stronger and safer position. Adjust the height of the safety pin in the cage accordingly.

You will be working only the top 1/2 to 2/3 of the range of motion. Why limit the range of motion?—First, because you have already trained the bottom of the ROM with partial HLRs on a bar. Second, according to specialists from the former Soviet Union, the first 40-45 degrees of the HLR work the legs more than the abs.[55] Third, supine leg raises are hard on the back and not the abs.[56] Fourth, because I was extremely impressed with the effects of partial HLRs—L-seat to the top—when I spent a few months training under Ivan Ivanov, formerly one of the coaches for the Bulgarian National Gymnastics Team.

As before, you will start from the top, from full contraction. Get to the bar the safe and easy way. Bend your knees all the way and bring your knees towards your chest. Straighten out your legs and touch the bar with your insteps. Stay.

Take a breath, push down on the bar, and Hardstyle breathe in a familiar series of hisses until you have blown out most of your air and hopefully cramped every muscle on the front of your body.

At the same time push your insteps hard through the bar, as if you are determined to leave bloody welts on your skin. This will build your strength to finish a real hanging leg raise.

Without releasing the tension or stopping to push down on the bar, lower your legs until they form a ninety degree angle with your body. Inhale into your stomach through your nose on the way down.

Pause in the "L-seat" momentarily while staying tight, then power back up without thinking about your breathing. When your insteps touch the bar, perform the familiar series of hisses. I got the idea of forceful exhalation on the top of the HLR from a book by Dr. Michael Colgan and it has made a powerful difference in my training.

Do 3-5 sets of 3-5 reps of this exercise with 3-5min of rest between them. Do not forget to stretch. Train three times a week alternating this floor drill and the partial hanging leg raise. Say "See you later" to Hardstyle sit-ups for the time being.

Let us work on a subtle advanced technique of "manipulating space in the body" in order to achieve greater strength and flexibility. Old time strongmen loved tearing chains by expansion of their ribcages. Modern girevoy sport competitors drive kettlebells off their chests in the jerk by explosively opening their chests. You are going to do the opposite of this action to make your HLR stronger.

Imagine that your torso has been spray painted with red paint. Now finish your supine leg raise in such a manner that every spot on the front, from your armpits to your pelvis, has gotten darker. This can only happen when the same amount of paint is spread over a smaller surface. The surface of your skin will shrink when your muscles, some visible and some not, shorten. Your six-pack, external and internal obliques, TVA, serratus, internal intercostals, lats, pecs, major and minor... You don't need to be an expert anatomist, just contract—shorten—whatever you can.

It is logical that if you aim to minimize the space in the front of the torso, you want to maximize it on the back side. While the front contracts to blood red, the back stretches to pink. (It is a good thing that it is on your back and you don't have to look at it. Pink is a weak color. There is research showing that looking at it even briefly reduces your grip strength.)

Flexing the spine is not enough, your shoulder blades need to separate and give you a hump. This happens to be the job of the serratus anterior, the cool looking rib like muscles above your obliques. They are not just for looks though. The serratus has several functions, discussing which is outside the scope of this book, but the fact that it is informally known as the "boxer's muscle" should tell you that any self-respecting hard Comrade ought to train it. Indeed, one of the serratus' jobs is rolling the shoulder forward during a knockout cross. When you push down on the bar in the HLR, obviously you are not using your arms only; the serratus is a major player.

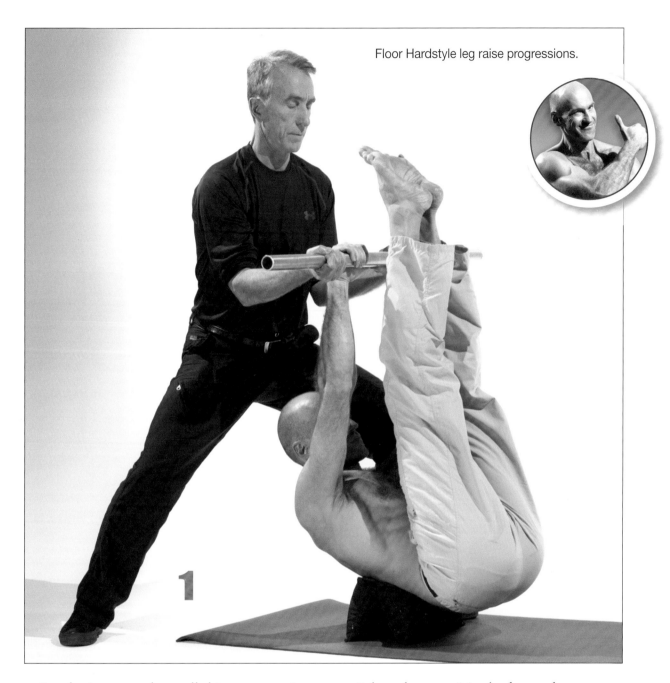

Floor Hardstyle leg raise progressions.

But don't worry about all this anatomy, just try to "close the space" in the front of your torso when your insteps are pushing through the bar and forcefully expelling your air. On every set pick a different spot on the front of your torso and give it special attention.

At some point you will be comfortably doing sets of five reps. Stay there for several sessions and try to get a greater contraction every time.

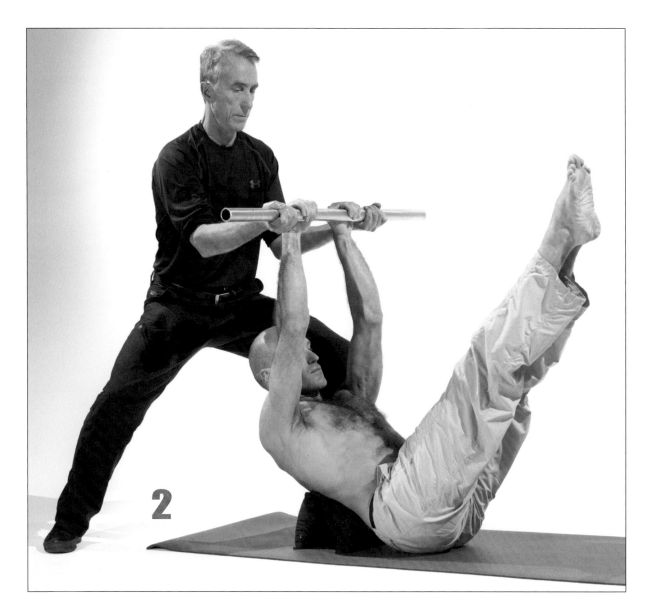

2

Then progress to the next level by slightly elevating your shoulders above your hips. You will need to place some heavy object—your training partner's feet and knees will do—behind you to prevent you from sliding. You will also need to move the pin up. Note that I don't yet want you to bring yours arms in line with your ears as they will be when you are hanging on the bar yet; for now stay with the easier partially closed (extended) shoulder.

At this angle you will be getting less help from gravity. Eventually progress to the point where you are sitting upright—but with the bar still slightly in front and not directly overhead.

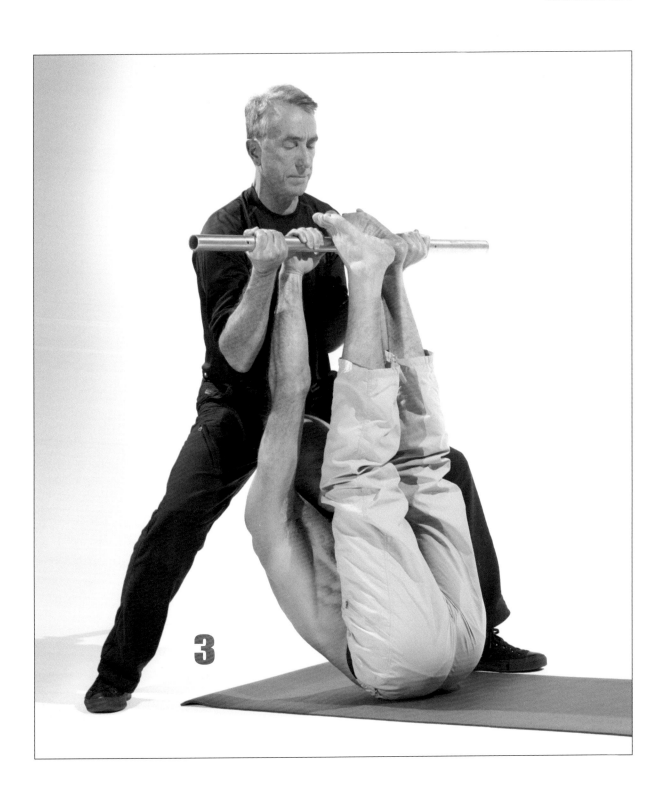

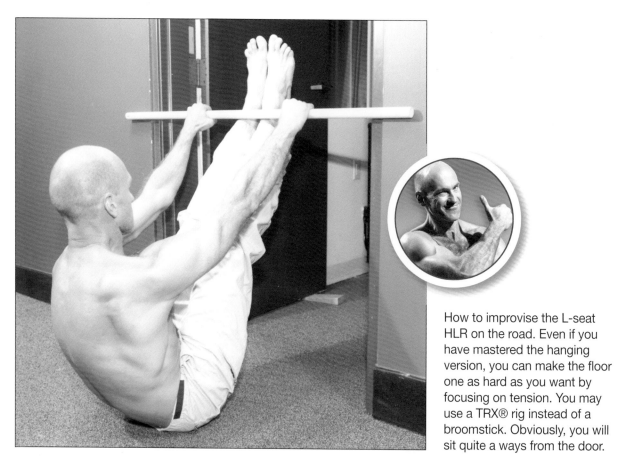

How to improvise the L-seat HLR on the road. Even if you have mastered the hanging version, you can make the floor one as hard as you want by focusing on tension. You may use a TRX® rig instead of a broomstick. Obviously, you will sit quite a ways from the door.

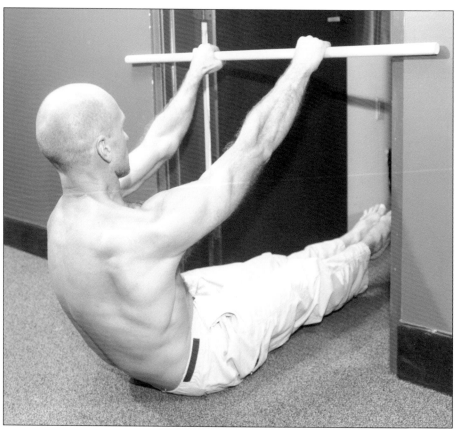

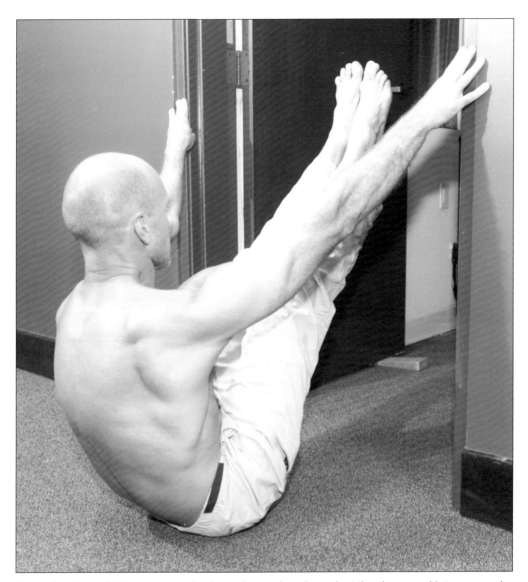

If no stick is available you may simply push your hands against the doorway. Not everyone's shoulders will like it.

You are ready to graduate to the "real" hanging leg raise. You already know how to do it, you just need to learn one subtlety concerning the negative.

On the way down reengage the glutes—contract them—when your legs have almost reached the L-seat position. This will make the bottom half of the exercise more intense while unloading your back.

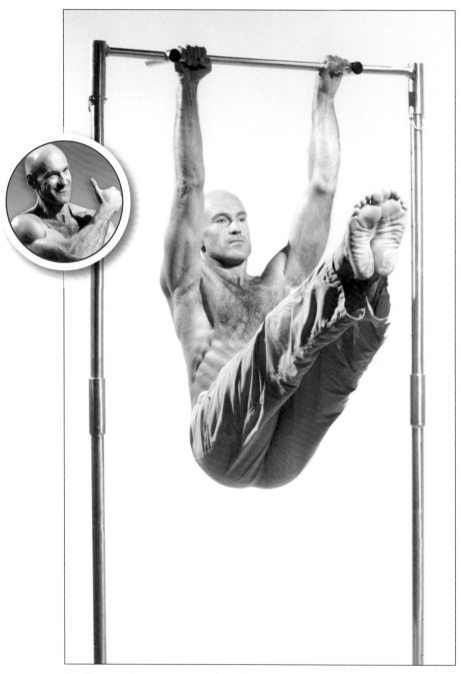

On the way down reengage the glutes at this point.

On the bottom, as in Hardstyle sit-ups, you have two options. Either stay tight and power back up. Or relax completely, let your bad breath out, and allow your spine stretch for a second before inhaling and reengaging the tension for the next rep.

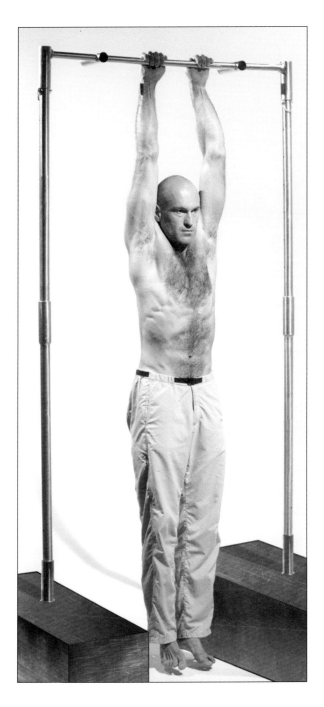
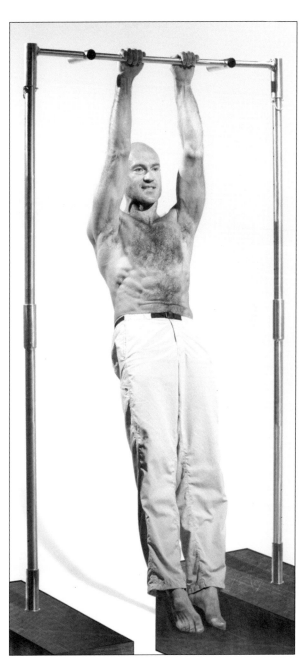

Loose or tight: two ways to separate your reps.

You can bring some variety into your HLR training by changing your grip. In addition to the narrow thumbless grip use the shoulder width grip with the thumbs around the bar. Do not forget the parallel narrow grip either. Rif is a big fan of HLRs on rings, as this piece of equipment gives the shoulders the freedom to move the way they wish to.

As you get stronger, consider the following more advanced HLR variations. Remember to Hardstyle breathe and cramp everything on the top of each rep.

1) HLR touching the bar with the shins, instead of the insteps. According to Dr. Ivan Belsky, sports scientist and elite strength coach, this variation maximally engages the abs.

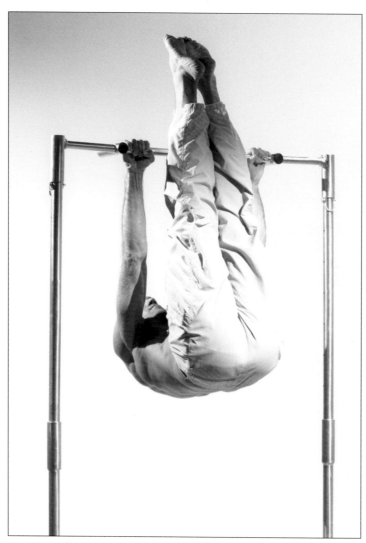

HLR touching the bar with the shins.

2) Top half HLR, from the L-seat to the top and back.

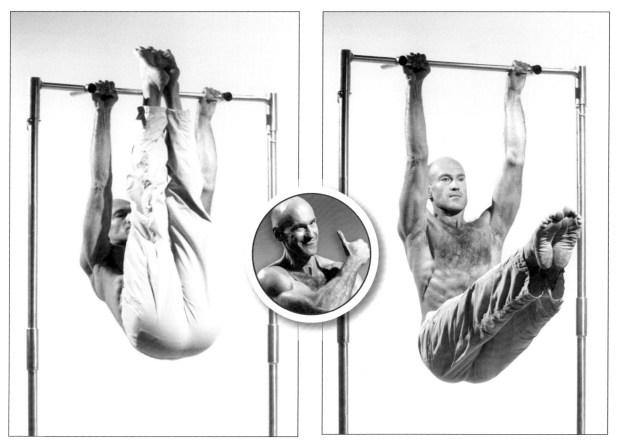

Top half HLR.

3) Top half HLR with pauses in the L-seat. "Back in the primordial days of yore," wrote Marty Gallagher on the subject of paused lifts, "men sought to make lifts more difficult: nowadays men seek ways to make lifts easier. We resurrect this ancient philosophy of making *resistance* training hard—ponder the irresolvable contradiction of making *resistance* training *easier*."

Ivan Ivanov had me do the following nasty: (1sec L-seat hold + 1 rep), (2sec L-seat hold + 2 reps), etc., all the way up to 10 (I had to be helped towards the end). This is way too many reps for the Hardstyle plan, but you get the idea. Something like three reps with 3sec holds will do the trick.

Pausing on the top, pressing the insteps through the bar for a few seconds, is another option. Combining pauses at the top and in the L-seat is even better. You may also introduce pauses at both mid and top positions of a full range HLR.

4) HLR with ankle weights. The author of excellent book ***Building the Gymnastic Body,*** Chris Sommer comments: "Except for occasional forays to break up the monotony of training and some specialized equipment exercises, I do not train my athletes with high repetitions during physical preparation. I am far more interested in the generation of athletic power than I am in the development of endurance. The stronger and more powerful an athlete is, the higher the degree of athleticism they will be capable of exhibiting. To that end, I find that weighted leg lifts are the far more beneficial choice for future athletic excellence then endless high rep sets of the weightless variety."

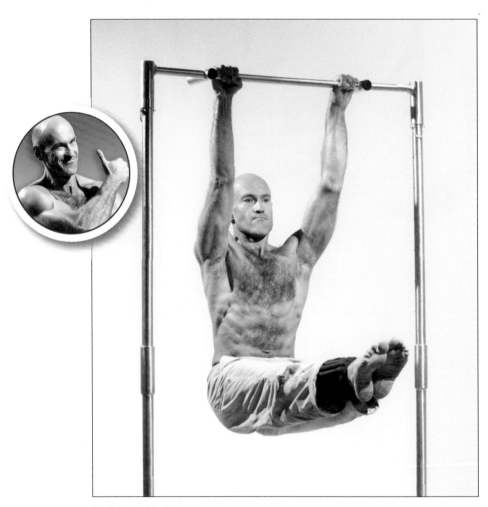

Weighted HLR.

5) Angled HLR. A simple way to make the HLR tougher and to challenge your external obliques more is to touch the bar with your shins not in the center but slightly—slightly!—outside one of the hands. This variation calls for the narrow grip.

The secret to the angled HLR is pulling harder with one arm—without bending either. Visualize your lats, pecs, serratus, and external obliques on the working side maximally shortening, closing your ribs, and bringing your pelvis and your ribs together on one side. A good way to implement this variation into your program is three way HLRs: left-right-straight for a triple or left-right-left-right-straight for a fiver.

Do not bother with "windshield wipers". They will not challenge your midsection but they will hurt your shoulders.

Do not attempt one-arm HLRs; it is a party trick, not an exercise. You will be too busy worrying about not ripping your shoulder out of the socket to work your abbies well.

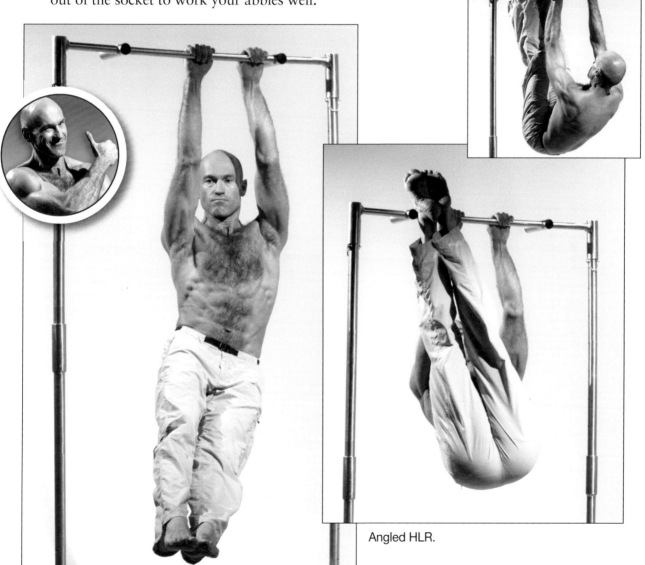

Angled HLR.

6) The Hardstyle HLR—Hardstyle breathing all the way. A friend of mine, an exceptionally strong man, called me up the day after I had him try the following version. "Were you trying to kill me? I did only three reps and I still feel my entire abdominal wall."

Normally you have hissed on the bottom, to take the slack out of the body, and the very top, to get a cramp, without worrying about your breathing in the middle. Now keep hissing all the way. It is evil.

Although it is the usual series of short hisses rather than one long hiss, do your best to make the movement of the legs smooth and not jerky. You may hiss on the negative as well. Do not think about inhalation, it will take care of itself as you will automatically "sip" air between hisses.

This variation is a form of internal isometrics; you can make it as hard as you wish.

Sissies hate the hanging leg raise because it is excruciatingly tough. It takes real strength in the waist and the lats, something the high rep crunch generation does not possess. It also takes flexibility and most muscle men are about as limber as astronauts in Moon suits. You have two choices. You could keep whining about how hard it is to hold on to the bar, how much your shoulders hurt, and how you do not feel anything in your abs. Or, you could rise up to the challenge. The bar is set high and it is waiting.

FOOTNOTES

46 Bret Contreras' data

47 "RA, EO and TrA act at optimal force-generating length in the midrange of lumbar spine flexion, where IO can generate approximately 90% of its maximum force." (Brown et. al, 2010)

48 Monfort (1998), Bankoff & Furlina (1984)

49 Tarnanen et al. (2008)

50 Kendall et. al (1971) point out that normally downward movement of the arms, or shoulder extension "requires fixation by abdominal muscles. [However,] when abdominal weakness exists, however, fixation for the downward pull or push of the arm may be provided by the back muscles. For example, if a patient is placed in a supine position and given resistance to a downward pull of both arms, normal abdominal muscles will contract to fix the thorax firmly toward the pelvis. However, if extensive abdominal weakness is present, the back will arch from the table, and the thorax will pull away from the pelvis until it is firmly fixed by extension of the thoracic spine. The arching of the back stretches the abdominal muscles, and they may appear firm under tension. The examiner must be careful not to mistake this tautness for firmness due to actual contraction of the muscles."

51 "*Bilateral weakness of external obliques decreases* the ability to flex the vertebral column and tilt the pelvis posteriorly… The posterolateral fibers of the external oblique are elongated as the thoracic spine flexes during the trunk curl. These fibers of the external oblique help to draw the posterior rib cage toward the anterior iliac crest, and in so doing, they tend to extend, not to flex, the thoracic spine…" (Kendall et al., 2005)

52 "Weakness of the external oblique is common in persons performing excessive sit-up exercises because the posterolateral fibers of the external oblique elongate during the trunk curl." (Kendall et al., 2005)

53 Chek (1992)

54 Ratov (1972, 1987, 1994), Yevseyev & Rykunov (1984)

55 Belsky (2003)

56 "The rectus abdominis muscle… is relatively inactive [in supine leg raises]; it secures the pelvis and increases the intraabdominal pressure. It begins to shorten only when the legs are raised high enough. At this point, however, the moment of force gravity, pulling the legs down, is relatively slight. Since the initial pressure on the discs is rather high and the activity of the abdominal wall muscles is not significant… this exercise is not especially valuable… Leg raising in a hanging position is much more effective (here the rectus abdominis contracts when the moment of gravity of the legs reaches its maximum), but it is feasible only for trained persons." (Zatsiorsky, 1995)

The Hardstyle Abs program design

> I NEVER WENT TO THE GYM TO "WORK OUT".
> RATHER I WENT TO LEARN.
> THE WORKOUT WAS INCIDENTAL.
> —DR. ED THOMAS

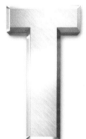People love making categorical statements like "The abs must be trained every day!", "The abs should never be trained every day!", "Train your abs three times a week", etc. Yes and no to all of the above. Strength coaches' experience tells us that a wide variety of schedules may work. For instance, powerlifting champions train their bench press anywhere between once and eight times a week—an enormous spread.

The individual frequency, volume, etc. depend on many variables. Start with the following cookie cutter recommendations, then adjust. I am not going to waste pages explaining the logic behind the following template. If you are familiar with my previous work, you already understand it. If you are not, remember that the Party is always right and follow the orders without questioning them.

- Treat your training session as a "practice"—not a "workout". Focus on maximizing the tension in different midsection muscles and linkage between them.

- Do not evaluate your progress by the number of reps you can do; as your tension skill improves, your rep count might drop. Instead, track your ability to perform more advanced versions of the given exercises or other challenging midsection exercises.

- Do not train your abs before heavy lifting or when you are tired. The ideal time is after a low volume strength workout or in a separate workout.

- It is safer to perform spine flexion exercises in the evening than in the morning.

- Train your midsection three times per week.

- Alternate two weeks of Hardstyle sit-ups and two weeks of leg raises (block training).

- Feel free to use different variations of the same exercise in different workouts (*specialized variety*).

  — E.g. Hardstyle sit-ups starting from the top on Monday, starting from the floor and relaxing between reps on Wednesday, "1 ½" reps on Friday.

- Perform 1-5 repetitions per set.

- Never train to failure. Stop when you still have 1-2 reps "in the bank".

- Do a total of 10-25 reps per session.

  — E.g. 5x2, 3x5, (2,3,5)x2, (1, 2, 3, 4, 5), etc.

- If greater hypertrophy is the goal, slowly increase this number to 50 in one of the weekly sessions.

  — E.g. 10x5 (sets x reps), (2, 3, 5)x5.

- The length of rest between the sets in minutes should approximately match the number of reps in the last set. You do not need a stopwatch, close enough is good enough. You may reduce these intervals when hypertrophy is the priority.

  — E.g. 2min of rest after 2 reps, 5min after 5 reps, etc.

- Stretch your abs and perform some easy non-related exercise during the rest intervals.

  — E.g., practice *Fast & Loose* drills, shadowbox, stretch your hips, foam roll your piriformis and IT bands, do some calf raises, etc.

  — I am a fan of the protocol by Steve Baccari, RKC: every couple of minutes alternate sets on the Ab Pavelizer™ and Captains of Crush® grippers. I do not know an easier way to significantly improve one's strength in almost any exercise and performance in almost any sport than heavy ab training plus heavy gripper training.

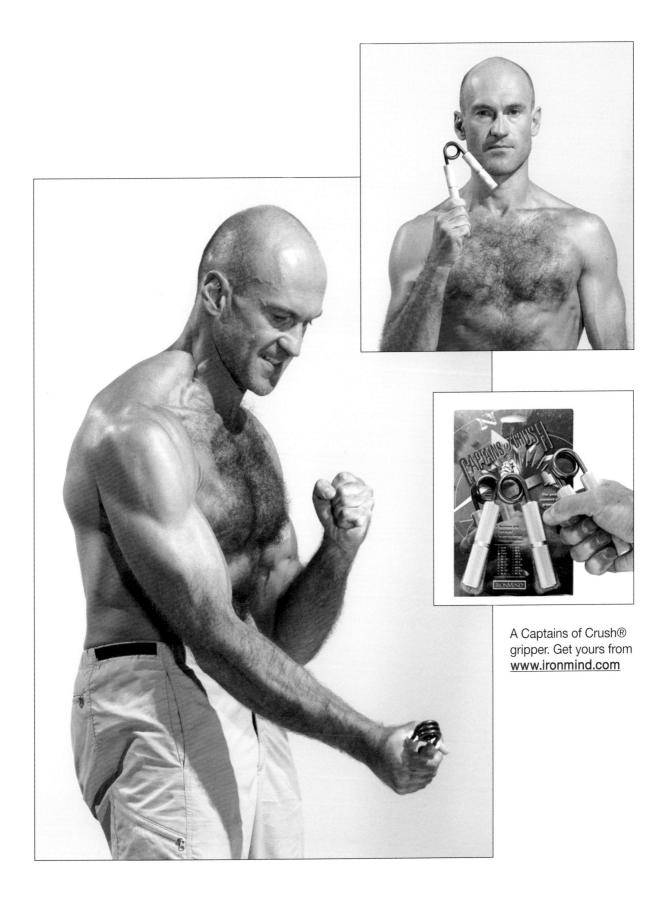

A Captains of Crush®
gripper. Get yours from
www.ironmind.com

- If you are short on time, you may divide your abdominal practice into two.

  — E.g. 2x5 in the morning and 3x5 in the evening.

- If you are unable to do your scheduled abdominal workout, practice Hardstyle breathing throughout the day.

- If you are on a high volume strength regimen, reduce or eliminate direct ab work.

  — *Enter the Kettlebell!* **Program Minimum**. Given the volume of get-ups, any sit-up work would be redundant. 10 HLRs twice a week on GU free days should not be a problem.

  — *Enter the Kettlebell!* **Rite of Passage**. One-arm military press ladders smoke the midsection. At most you should do a total of 10 reps of either Hardstyle sit-ups or HLRs on variety days. Or none at all.

  — *Return of the Kettlebell!*, *Kettlebell Muscle*, **Smolov Squat**, **Russian Squat Routine**. Don't even think about it.

  — *Power to the People!* The "Bear" will tolerate no direct ab work. On the other hand, the base PTP plan and *Hardstyle Abs* are fully compatible.

  — *The Naked Warrior.* 10 reps per workout twice a week of Hardstyle sit-ups or HLRs, as one-arm pushups are very demanding on the midsection.

- Follow the *Hardstyle Abs* plan twice a year for 8-12 weeks.

What should one do in the interim?—Heavy lifting.

Dr. Franco Columbu told me that he hated abdominal exercises. So he just focused on contracting his abs hard in every strength exercise—even the bench press. "Every exercise was about my abs!" Not only did he win the Mr. Olympia title, but the "Best Abs" award as well. Behold the power of high tension!

At a buck eighty Columbu deadlifted over 700 pounds. I hope you follow this old school bodybuilder's suit and never allow your physique goals to distract you from being strong.

Power to you!

Opposite and following page: Strong + lean = ripped
Photos courtesy Dr. Franco Columbu

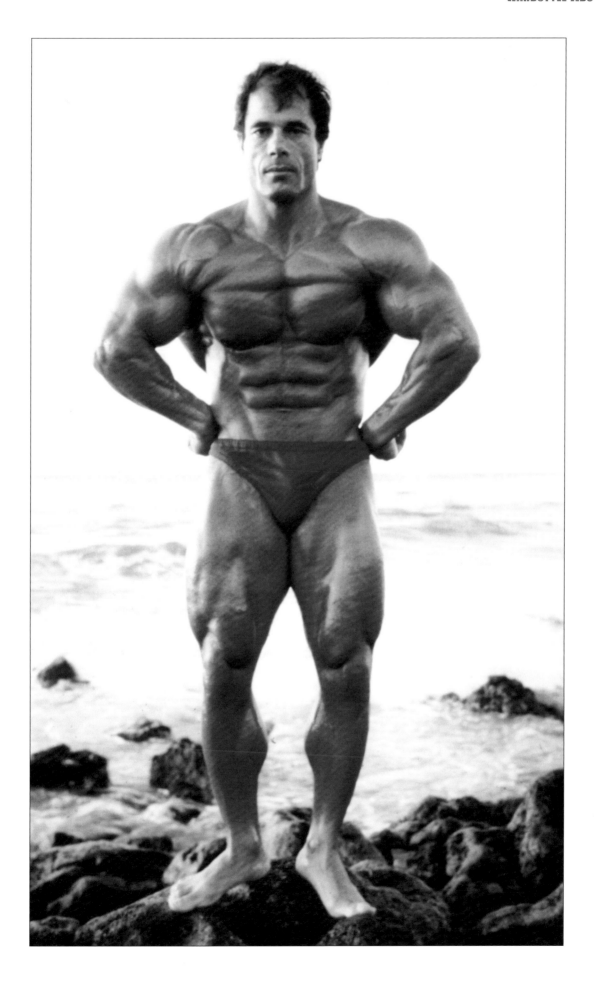

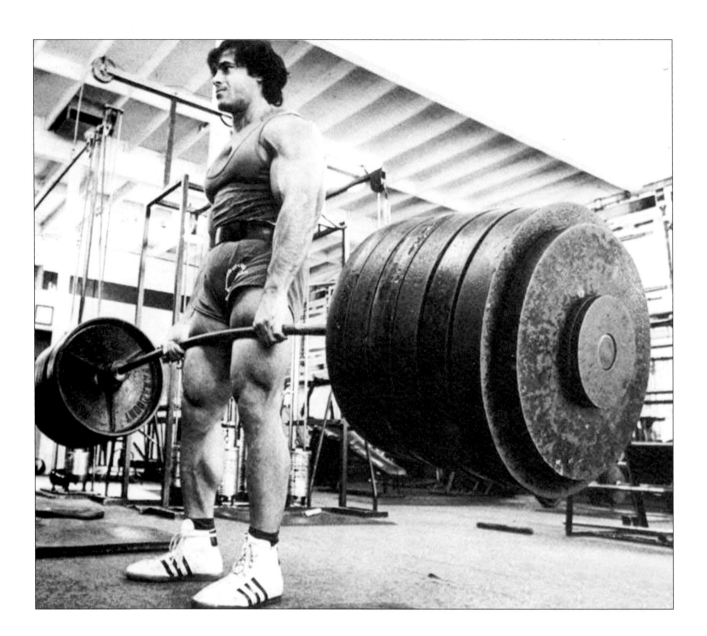

Appendix:
A few words about "functional core training"

I'VE NEVER MET A PERSON WITH A 300-POUND DEADLIFT THAT DIDN'T HAVE MORE CORE STRENGTH THAN ANY OF THESE PENCIL-NECKED FITNESS EXPERTS WHO ENDLESSLY PROCLAIM THE MYSTICAL BENEFITS OF MORE CORE.
—MARTY GALLAGHER

Functional training", as I understand it, is supposed to teach—or rather remind—one how to move like a Paleolithic hunter. It happens to be one of the goals of the Hardstyle methodology.

What we never do at Hardstyle is divorce movement from strength. We reject the circus clown exercises as taught by personal trainers across the fruited plain. We subscribe to the FT philosophy of Gray Cook, the physical therapist of choice for the NFL and the Navy SEALs. These hard men know with their guts that "functional" cannot belong in the same sentence with "weak".

Ironically, without strength, there is no good movement. "A heavy weight reveals the biomechanical truth behind an exercise," quipped former Senior RKC Rob Lawrence. The "un-Cooked" FT folks do not "move authentically", they are just faking it. A couple of years ago my friend Marty Gallagher wrote an article titled "Doing Fewer Things Better" which drove a stake through their hearts:

In the big fat world of fitness, things keep getting ever more crazed. The general fitness clientele, to expropriate a musical analogy, are dazed and confused. I keep seeing whacky stuff on TV as personal trainers will do anything to differentiate themselves from other personal trainers…how about sitting on the infamous Swiss Ball, one leg extended as the other fights to maintain balance while pushing a tiny-weenie dumbbell overhead. The only thing missing is circus music and perhaps a mini-car circling the exercising trainee that suddenly stops as eight clowns pile out. Meanwhile a muscle-less "fitness expert" dramatically intones that doing the overhead dumbbell press (with a weight my 90-pound daughter could rep a dozen times) while fighting for balance "builds core strength." It seems that every crackpot exercise shown as of late builds that elusive core strength…gimme some core strength…gotta have that core strength….of course I've never met a person with a 300-pound deadlift that didn't have more core strength than any of these pencil-necked fitness experts who endlessly proclaim the mystical benefits of more core. These experts keep insisting and proscribing that their clients need more core strength; it's become the predictable mantra of the new age fitness world. Here's a flash bulletin: achieving a 150-pound pause squat taken below parallel for 10-reps will infuse more core strength then all the Swiss Ball sit-ups, presses and off-balanced dink-ass exercises combined. That's a natural fact: mathematically irrefutable and demonstrable.

…Let's get off the Swiss Balls waving tiny dumbbells too insignificant to trigger hypertrophy, let's stop substituting sub-maximal effort and feeling good about ourselves for substantive physical progress, let's stop pretending and start actualizing, let's get freaking serious and that means stripping away all the toys and distractions and get back to bold basics. Let's start mastering basic fitness themes before spinning off into all the cute little variations that net nothing.

"Heavy weight is instructive," states Cook. Take some rotary movement like the full contact twist. Even if the student succeeds in keeping a neutral spine, locking his rib cage to his pelvis, and not moving his shoulders and he moves at a controlled cadence, as he should, he will not learn anything about transferring force from the ground up into his hands until the weight on the bar gets noticeable by the given exercise's standards, e.g. a 45-pound plate for a 180-pound man. It takes a heavy weight to line up the vectors of force and to adequately stiffen the linkage. You will never understand this until you have been under heavy iron. "A heavy weight teaches with a big stick," promises Gallagher.

A heavy weight is a good teacher—provided it is moved slowly. And please don't feed me any indignant non-sense about "only fast being functional". If you cannot do something slow, you have no right to do it fast. With some exceptions, failure to do a movement slowly indicates that you, as Gray puts it, "are hiding something". A compensation, a weakness. Which is why our get-up master Dr. Mark Cheng, Senior RKC often has his students practice get-ups at "Tai Chi speed". Incidentally, he has his martial arts students do the same with kicks. One gets to cram a lot of physics and skill and identify his problem areas when momentum is no longer an option. No wonder kickboxing legend Bill "Superfoot" Wallace made slow kicks an essential element of his championship practice.

As a rule of thumb, in Hardstyle exercises we move slower or faster than comfortable in order to get the most benefits. For instance, we slow down our get-ups and speed up our swings.

Another problem with the "un-Cooked" is, they fail to resolve some more fundamental mobility problems before practicing the primal patterns. For instance, in order to achieve a perfect deep squat in a way that does not gun the gas pedal against the parking brakes and set one up for a hip replacement surgery down the road, the person must have a flexible pelvic floor. Only when the sit-bones spread apart, can the hip joints move freely into the squat. A rigid pelvic floor prevents such separation and grinds the femoral heads.

Hence most squats out there are labored and "non-authentic". Trainers have their clients do all sorts of fancy stretches for the muscles surrounding the hip joints and foam roll, yet as they do not recognize that the pelvis can and should separate, they fail. In the Hardstyle system, in contrast, we stretch the pelvic floor and teach the student to distract the hips and find freedom in his body while we are teaching him to squat. A Hardstyle squat looks natural and effortless as you learn to get out of your own way. (This is the Yin of stretching and opening space to the Yang of tension and compactness.) And we do it without big words and fancy contraptions.

Senior RKC and *Black Belt* columnist Dr. Mark Cheng adds: "True Hardstyle is built on a platform of fundamental elasticity and mobility. Generating extreme tension without the reactive ability to "take the brakes off" when needed is little more than developing rigid, awkward movement and fooling yourself into thinking that it's stability. A functional athlete has developed the skill of dynamic motor control, using strength in all the right places, at all the right times, and tested its maximal weight."

To return our "functional training" discussion to the "core", planks are worse than worthless if one has tight hip flexors and atrophied glutes. The trainee will end up reinforcing the pattern of using his hip flexors as the core. Hardstyle sit-ups and hip flexor stretches from *Hardstyle Abs* rewire one to plank right. As we do at the RKC kettlebell instructor course. Physiologist Bret Contreras took EMG measurements to compare the peak activation of various midsection muscles in the traditional front plank and the RKC version and here are the results:

Exercise	Lower Rectus Abdominis (RA)	Internal Oblique (IO)	External Oblique (EO)
Standard Plank	33.5	42.6	26.7
RKC Plank	115.0	99.5	104.0

In the RKC plank the lower abs contracted more than three times more intensely, the internal obliques more than twice, the external obliques almost four times as intensely as in the typical plank seen in gyms everywhere. Because we pay attention to detail. For instance, we teach maximal pelvic floor activation. Just as extreme flexibility demands that the PF stretches, extreme strength demands that it contracts. We teach Hardstyle breathing and other key strength skills. When we are done with you, you are ready to plank, if this is what you want to do.

You will also be ready for various "functional" exercises that require one to move against a load in different planes while maintaining a stiff torso and a neutral spine. Prof. Stuart McGill[57] took EMG measurements of several such drills. For instance, in the "cable walkout" the subjects grabbed the cable in both hands and then walked sideways. The RA showed a measly 10% peak activation and the EO did not quite make it to 25%. The IO managed to squeak past 70% MVC, but that is not surprising as any heavy exertion brings these muscles "online" in people with normal firing patterns.

The premier spine biomechanist observed that "the muscle activation levels were modest even though the tasks were quite strenuous..." He explained that "single muscles cannot be activated to 100% MVC in these whole-body standing exercises that do not isolate joints. This is because most torso muscles create movements about the 3 orthopedic axes of the spine. If a muscle were activated to a higher level, unwanted movements would occur that would have not be balanced by other muscles. This places a constraint on the activation level of any muscle in a 'functional exercise'." McGill concluded that, "Perhaps these constraints are one aspect of what separates "functional" exercises from muscle isolationist exercises..."

In other words, stuff like that might teach you a thing or two about movement but it will not make you strong. In my opinion, such exercises are the domain of physical therapists and corrective specialists. Half-kneeling chops are great but you need to know what you are chopping and why.

One "functional" exercise I recommend to anyone and to which I am not surprisingly partial is the kettlebell get-up. Steve Maxwell introduced it to RKC years ago and since then RKC heavyweights Gray Cook, Dr. Mark Cheng, Brett Jones, and Jeff O'Connor have dug "a mile deep" into this remarkable exercise. The GU's benefits and applications could fill a book.

Cook comments, "The Turkish Get-Up is the perfect example of training primitive movement patterns—from rolling over, to kneeling, to standing and reaching. If I were limited to choosing only one exercise to do, it'd be the Turkish Get-Up. This is the only exercise that honors the entire Functional Movement Screen."

"For many athletes learning to lock the ribcage on the pelvis is essential for injury prevention and performance..." stresses McGill. "[A] terrific exercise for transitioning into performance is the Turkish Getup, where the spine posture is controlled and the overhead weight is steered as the body learns more movement strategies that maintain torso stiffness while driving with other extremities."

"The kettlebell community has praised the core-activating benefits of the Turkish Get Up for many years," writes Bret Contreras. "It's taken quite a while for some strength coaches to catch on but nowadays most coaches are having their athletes perform the TGU in their warm-ups. The TGU was the only exercise [out of fifty-two] in this experiment that had over 100% peak activation in all four core muscles that were tested. Good job, kettlebellers!"

The physiologist got these surprisingly high readings and it only took a fifty-pounder:

Exercise	Lower RA	IO	EO	Lumbar Erector
50lb. Get-Up	133.0	138.0	191.0	139.0

It must be noted that if you choose to use the GU as your only source of developing rock hard abs, it will take considerable volume. While the peak activation of each midsection muscle is very high, the mean activation is modest, in the 30-40% range. Neither muscle fires this hard for a long time as the athlete keeps changing the direction of loading. You will have to punch in more reps to have more time under high tension for each muscle. We do just that in the *Enter the Kettlebell!* Program Minimum.

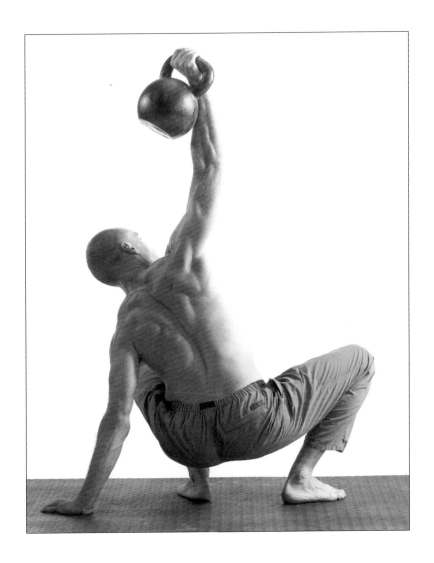

FOOTNOTES

57 McGill et al. (2009)

Appendix:
Full contact abs

ALWAYS THINK CONSCIOUSLY OF THE FACT
THAT THE STRENGTH FOR EVERY TECHNIQUE
COMES FROM THE HARA.
—A. PFLUGER, *KARATE BASIC PRINCIPLES*

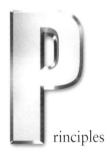rinciples

Fighters' midsections must to do five things well.

1. *Act as body armor.*

2. *Transfer the power between the lower and the upper body without energy losses and with good spine mechanics.*

3. *Maintain proper breathing behind braced abs for the duration of the fight (Yin breathing).*

4. *Explosively compress the breath and to stiffen up the body on impact (Yang breathing).*

5. *Provide reflexive rotary stability.*

The first item is the most obvious one. Hypertrophy of the abdominal wall is in order. Up the number of sets of Hardstyle sit-ups and hanging leg raises to thicken the six-pack. Chad Waterbury, strength coach for Ralek Gracie and director of strength and conditioning for the Rickson Gracie International Jiu-Jitsu Academy, comments:

> When it comes to training fighters, using nothing but planks and similar exercises that focus on developing core tension while maintaining a neutral spine isn't optimal. Your nervous system always knows the best way to protect yourself—that's its job. If someone throws a front kick toward your gut, the reflex action is to pull the ribcage down to develop maximal tension in the abdominals. The high-tension reaction serves to protect your organs like a plate of armor. This reflex action is hardwired into your nervous system, much like the hip flexion withdrawal when you step on a tack. No one lifts his chest or pushes his stomach out when a strike is coming towards his midsection because the nervous system knows better. For abdominal tension to reach its peak, drawing the ribcage down toward the pelvis is necessary and this is accompanied by some degree of spinal flexion. Full spinal flexion should never be the goal when training the core, or any other exercise, since it's almost always best to maintain lordosis. However, a fighter must develop his ability to quickly induce high levels of abdominal tension in order to withstand strikes to the midsection, and this requires the amount of spinal flexion necessary to pull his ribcage down. Any spinal flexion beyond what it takes to pull your ribcage down is unnecessary and high-risk to your spine.

The sides are effectively built up with full contact twists, suitcase deadlifts, and various Zercher lifts. Hanging leg raises will go a long way as well.

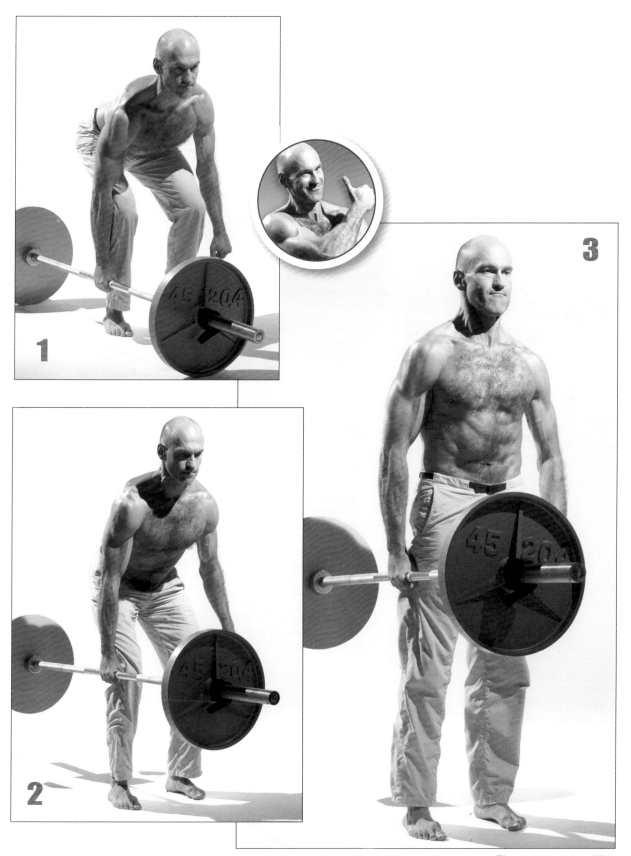

The suitcase deadlift.

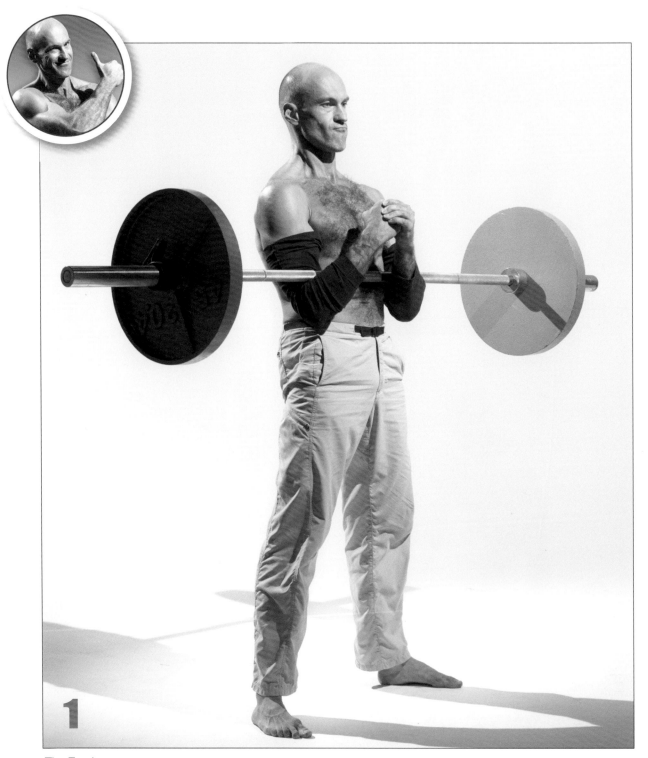

1

The Zercher squat.

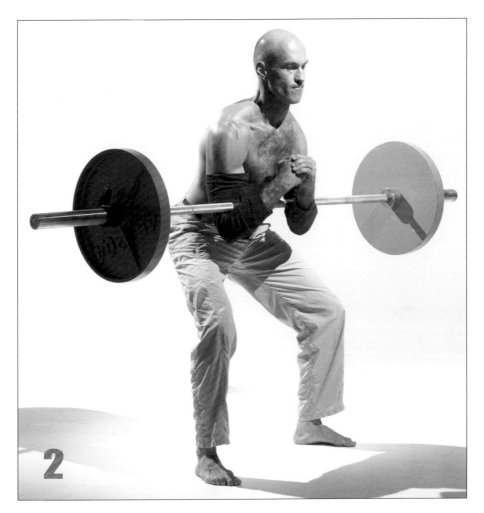

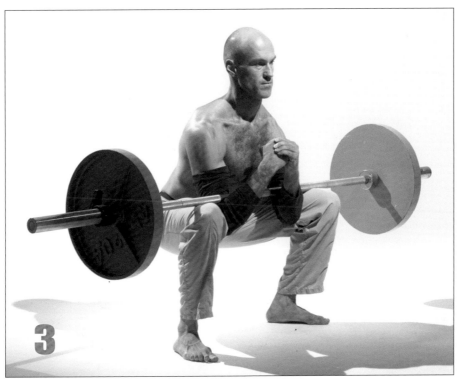

For the second item the drill of choice is the full contact twist, which I will describe in a minute. As a thrower, a fighter ought to do low sets of low reps, e.g. 3-5x3-5, not the typical high rep nonsense (we will discuss building muscular endurance the right way in #3). In the immortal words of elite MMA strength coach Steve Baccari, RKC, "Before working on strength endurance you need to have some strength to endure."

Norwegian scientists conducted two studies, one on long distance runners[58] and the other on cyclists[59]. These experienced endurance athletes were put on a pure strength program, 4x4RM half-squats three times a week, in addition to their usual endurance training. Eight weeks later the athletes not only got stronger and more explosive—without gaining any weight!—they improved endurance in their sport: their movement efficiency improved and the time they could last to exhaustion at maximal aerobic power increased.

On the energy systems continuum—alactacid, lactacid, aerobic—throwers are on one extreme end of the spectrum, with long distance runners and bicyclists are on the other, and fighters in the middle. Would it not be logical that if low rep pure strength training helped pure endurance athletes, it would help you even more? As a bonus, such training is non-exhaustive and, as you have seen, it does not increase one's bodyweight.

How does it work?—The stronger the muscle, the less it has to contract to produce a given amount of force.[60] It may be obvious, but it is profound. In the above studies the athletes increased their movement economy and decreased their perceived effort. How does our body perceive effort?

The nervous system measures the intensity of the neural drive going to the muscles.[61] The muscles send back messages about the level of tension generated, the speed of movement, and the distance covered. The brain compares the intensity of the "nerve force" with the outcome and determines the degree of effort.[62] In other words, how much bang (mechanical work) do you get for the buck (the intensity of the "nerve force"). A weight may "feel" heavy not because it is heavy but because it takes a lot of "juice" to move it.

"The size of the neural drive required to generate a given external force is influenced by a number of factors, but principally by the force-generating capacity of the muscle. A strong muscle requires a lower neural drive to generate a given force, because the force represents a smaller proportion of its maximum capacity. Similarly, a fatigued muscle requires a higher neural drive to generate a given force, because the force represents a higher proportion of its maximum capacity."[63]

Which is why a strong fighter who is skilled enough at relaxation can go the distance: he is barely trying and still putting out a heck of a power. This applies to all your muscles, with those of the midsection being a special case.

Prof. Stuart McGill explains:

Storage of elastic energy in a compliant spring, or a soft spring is rapidly dissipated or lost. This happens if the muscle is not activated to a sufficient level. If the spring is too stiff, elastic energy storage is hampered because there is minimal elasticity and no movement... So, the pre-contraction level of the muscle just prior to the loading phase is extremely important... a lot of stiffness and stability is achieved in the first 25% of the maximum contraction level. From our work examining several different rapid loading situations, it appears that a pre-contraction level of about 25% MVC [maximal voluntary contraction] creates the amount of muscle stiffness for optimal storage and recovery of elastic energy in the core muscles (at least in many situations). Less than this results in a spongy system while more than this creates stiffness that impedes energy return and also unnecessarily crushes the spine and the joints.

It is a fact that tensing the midsection spreads tension all over the body—the phenomenon of *irradiation* I have written about in **Power to the People!** Which is great at the moment of the strike's impact but decidedly bad in flight. Russian full contact karate master and Spetsnaz vet Andrey Kochergin explains that rigidity is often the result of trying to lead the limb along its trajectory instead of letting it fly. He stresses: "Throw [the limb], then make an accent [*kime*] when it has arrived." One of his recommendations is relaxation training—"throw relaxed arms in different ways and in all directions and shake them until 'meat separates from the bones'"—but he also does heavy powerlifting training.

Only a strong person is able to stay truly relaxed when striking. If your abbies are weak, two equally unpleasant scenarios will play out.

One, you have managed to stay relaxed, in which case your soft underbelly will absorb a good part of your leg drive instead of passing it on to the shoulder ("You can't push a rope", famously quipped McGill). That means a weak strike.

Or two, you have stiffened your core enough—but it took so much effort that the tension has overflowed to your limbs. The punch is no longer a punch but a push, slow and tiring.

Having killer abs strengthened with low rep work will allow you to keep your torso stiffened just the right amount without even trying. Your limbs will stay relaxed, you will be powerful and not tired.

Now that I have hopefully convinced you to go heavy and do low reps, here is the drill.

The best exercise for transferring the hip power into the shoulder with a high interest is the full contact Twist. This exercise was originally developed in the Soviet Union for throwers. The then nameless twist came to fighters' attention when a famous Russian shot putter failed to talk his way out of a mugging. This mild mannered man got annoyed when one of the attackers cut him with a blade and he ruptured the punk's spleen with a single punch. Soviet justice's modus operandi could have been "Not a single good deed will go unpunished." But this time the innocent man defending his life got acquitted of manslaughter. The story made the papers.

One of the Comrades who read it was Igor Sukhotsky, formerly a nationally ranked weightlifter and an eccentric sports scientist who took up full contact Kyokushinkai karate at the age of forty-five. This renaissance man researched shot putters' training and noticed that the twist had not only increased his striking power, but also had toughened his midsection against blows. Sukhotsky was so impressed with the full contact twist that he added it to his super abbreviated strength training routine that consisted of only four exercises, the three powerlifts plus good mornings. It was Sukhotsky who popularized this drill among Russian fighters.

Load a barbell on one side. A hundred pound plate on the end of the bar is a reasonable goal for a serious athlete, but be sensible and start with a Barbie plate or an empty bar. Stick the other end in the corner. Protect the wall with a folded towel.

Pick up the loaded end of the bar and hold it in front of you with your fingers interlocked. The bar should be at approximately 45 degrees from the floor, although you may have to adjust the angle to suit your height and leverage.

Pick up the loaded end of the bar and hold it in front of you with your fingers interlocked. The bar should be at approximately 45 degrees from the floor, although you may have to adjust the angle to suit your height and leverage.

Setting up for the FCT.

Maintain a neutral spine for the duration of the set: avoid flexion, extension, or rotation.

Keep your arms straight and your knees slightly bent. If you have a hard time keeping your elbows locked, concentrate on flexing your triceps. It helps if you are a pistol shooter: the push-pull action of the straight arms is identical.

Remaining upright, inhale and turn the weight to one side while holding your breath. Don't lean with the bar, or away from the bar.

Pivot on your toes at the same time to avoid shearing forces on your knees. Make sure to wear shoes that do not catch on the surface where you are exercising. Even better, train barefoot.

Reverse the movement by tightening up your midsection and rotating your hips. Do not lift with your arms and shoulders. Do not exhale until you reach the top of the lift.

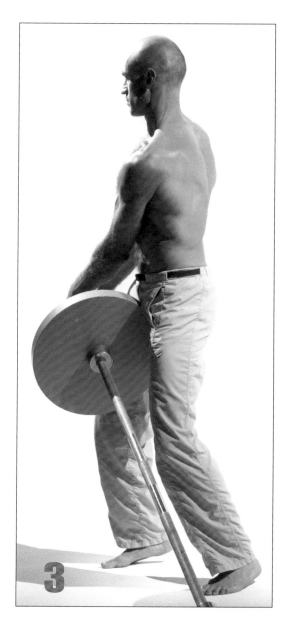
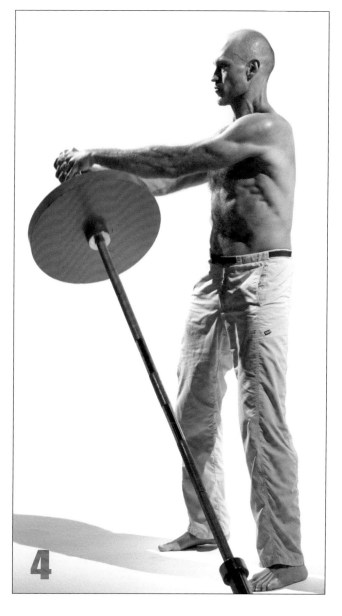

Control the weight at all times, don't use momentum.

Repeat the exercise in the opposite direction. That was one rep. You will need to readjust your stance slightly—you will figure out how when the weight gets heavy enough—when switching directions.

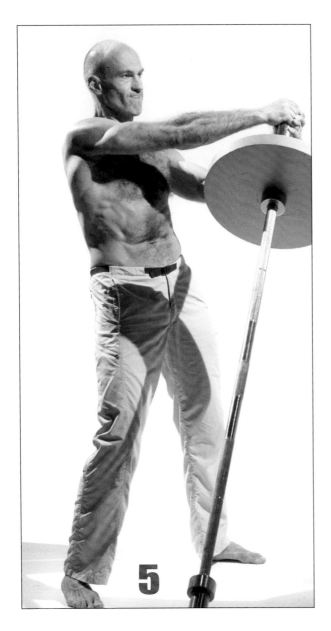
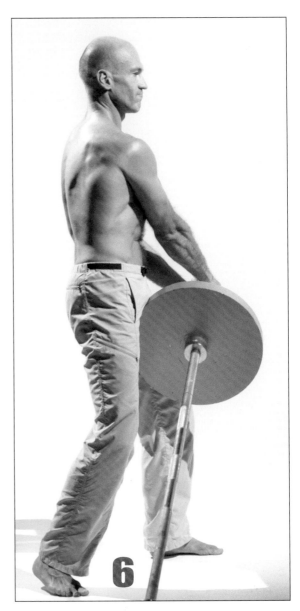

Now for the finer points. Do not lift the bar with your arms and shoulders. Initiate the twist with the ball of your right foot, then tense your right inner thigh. Contract your right glute and turn your hips to the left. Continue to your obliques and abs, compress your ribs, tense your lats, and only then move your rigid arms.

Let us go over the power chain one more time: the ball of the foot -> the inner thigh -> the glute -> the trunk -> the lats -> the arms -> the barbell.

This is a good time to state that in this "rotational" exercise there is no spine rotation: the ribcage is glued to the pelvis. When we tested the full contact twist at McGill's lab the professor was pleased to see that there was no spinal rotation involved. Something is twisting but that "something" is not the spine. McGill sums up: "The core, more often than not, functions to prevent motion rather than initiating it. Good technique in most sporting, and daily living tasks demands that power be generated at the hips and transmitted through a stiffened core."

3. Maintain proper breathing behind braced abs for the duration of the fight (Yin breathing).

This refers to not sucking wind and breathing with one's diaphragm when maintaining a brace or when the rib cage is restricted in ground fighting.

Sticking with traditional Asian terminology—"Ignoring the fundamentals of traditional karate is the gravest mistake"—Kancho Kochergin classifies martial breathing into "Yin breathing" and "Yang breathing". The former is used during wrestling, grappling, footwork, and some blocks. It is steady, even breathing punctuated by forced diaphragmatic exhalations during exertions: "breathing behind the shield". Wrestlers and grapplers, accustomed to long isometric contractions and restricted postures, have the advantage over strikers. It must be noted that Oriental martial arts have very sophisticated and effective variations of such breathing and a serious fighter owes it to himself to investigate them. And make sure to read the *Let Every Breath... Secrets of the Russian Breath Masters* book by Systema master Vladimir Vasiliev.

Prof. McGill comments on "Yin breathing": "An important feature of stable and functional backs is the ability to co-contract the abdominal wall independently of any lung ventilation patterns. Good spine stabilizers maintain the critical symmetric muscle stiffness during any combination of torque demand and breathing patterns... Training a breathing pattern to an exertion cycle may not be helpful."

The good professor, who unlike most of his colleagues, does not bother with "untrained college subjects" and prefers applying electrodes to great athletes like George St. Pierre, has developed an outstanding exercise to develop brace endurance and Yin breathing for fighters. He calls it "stir the pot". You will get to "integrate the entire anterior chain with torsional control".

Assume the front plank position with your forearms on an exercise ball. Look between your forearms, at the ball. Maintaining a neutral spine and steady breathing and not allowing the pelvis to move relative to the ribcage, start drawing progressively larger circles with your elbows. "Discipline is required for minimal spine motion but maximal shoulder motion," warns the scientist.

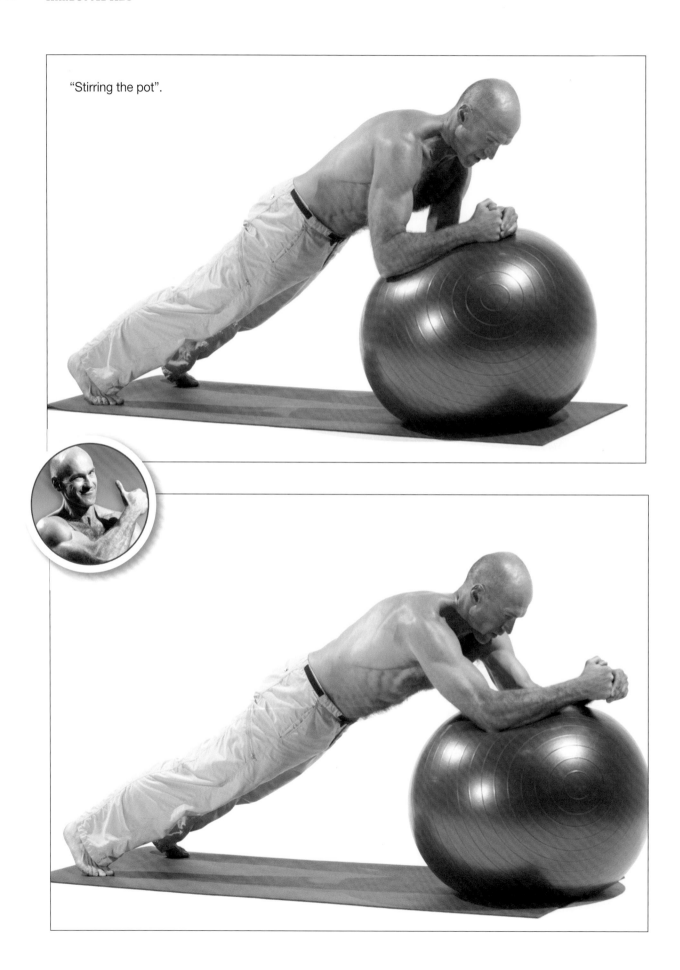

"Stirring the pot".

Stuart McGill recommends starting with multiple low rep sets and progressively building up to the duration of the fight, e.g. 5min followed by 1min of rest for MMA or multiple 2min rounds for kickboxing. He stresses that "the magic happens with maintaining breathing—diaphragm contraction/relaxation within the maintenance of the armor."

Another exercise worth considering, if it does not bother your back and your hamstrings are as flexible as they ought to be, is the L-seat hang on a pullup bar for time. As this is a "Yin exercise", don't use high tension techniques like gripping the bar, engaging the lats, or Hardstyle breathing. Breathe deep with your diaphragm and stay as relaxed as possible—without bending or dropping your legs or arching your lower back. The goal, according to Ivan Ivanov, formerly one of the coaches for the Bulgarian national gymnastics team, is 1min. Since this may not be long enough for a fighter and since I highly doubt that you will last even half that long, go straight to the "stir the pot" or the plank. Speaking of the latter, the goal Ivanov sets for the plank (tested when you are fresh) is 3min. (This is not the Yang plank with maximal tension for 10-20sec that we teach at the RKC course to develop tension for low rep strength exercises. This is the Yin plank where all the muscles contract at the same ratio but less intensely and the breathing is deep.)

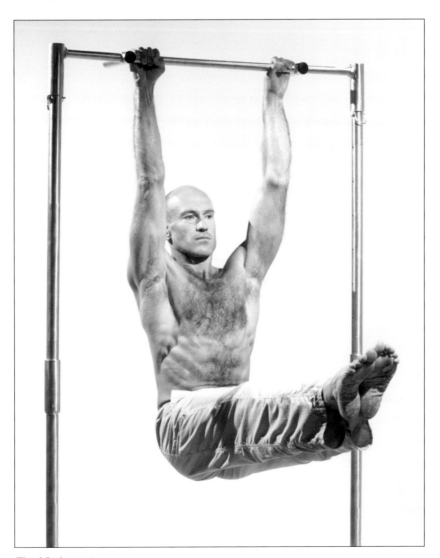

The Yin L-seat.

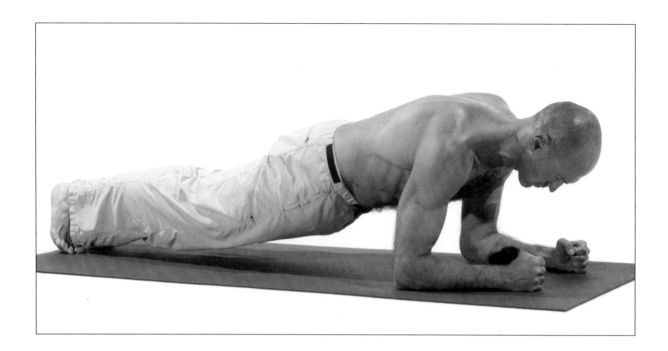

Russian full contact karate fighters do the following exercise to toughen up the body while practicing Yin breathing. Lie on your back, stretch your arms and legs out like a diver. Your sparring partner steps on you, while a third person holds his hand for balance. You start slowly rolling on the floor around the axis formed by your spine. At the same time your sparring partner is walking over your body with small steps. "A very hard exercise toughening the midsection and the torso muscles," promises Andrey Kochergin.

4. Explosively compress the breath and to stiffen up the body on impact (Yang breathing).

"Yang breathing" is breathing during a strike or some other explosive action. Unlike its Yin counterpart, it is synchronized with the movement, you "match your breath with the force". "A sharp exhalation is performed with maximal tension and ideally, for greater concentration, with a scream," comments Kochergin. "In the end of a Yang exhalation there is a breath hold, essential for instant concentration of a strike but counterproductive in long strength efforts of wrestling."

The following unique and simple exercise recommended by the authoritative Russian *Boxing Yearbook* will help you sharpen your Yang breathing while strengthening your punch—by developing a stronger and better timed fist and building forearm muscles. The author promises that this drill will work your muscles no less intensely than a barbell works a weightlifter's.

Get a large eraser or a rectangular block of rubber that comfortably fits into your fist, e.g. 1x1.5"x3". Carry it with you all day and squeeze it explosively. Initiate each gripping action from your *hara*—compress! Be maximally explosive—imagine that you are punching. Russian special operations hand-to-hand combat instructor V. Bykov has a helpful imagery: "Move and strike as if a grenade blew up inside you".

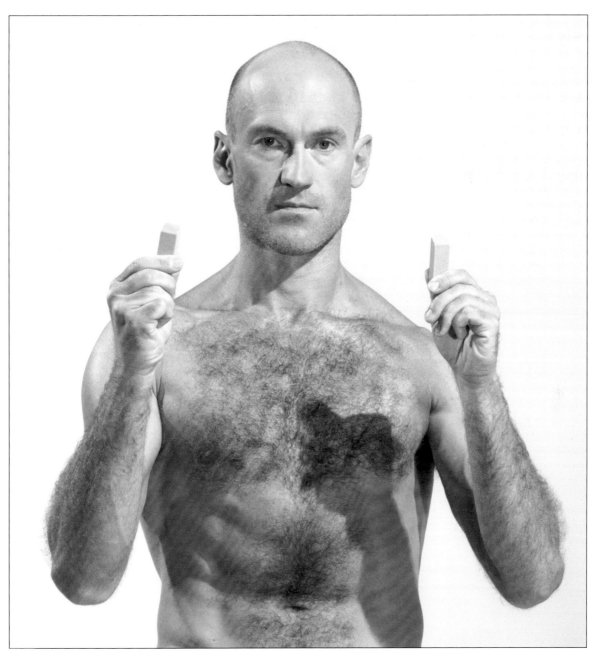

Get a large eraser or a rectangular block of rubber that comfortably fits into your fist. Carry it with you all day and squeeze it explosively.

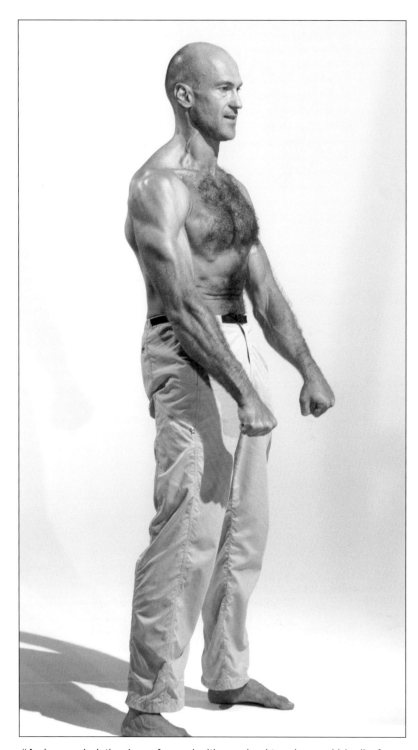

"A sharp exhalation is performed with maximal tension and ideally, for greater concentration, with a scream," comments Kochergin.

Then relax just as quickly as you have flexed! An expression by a famous Soviet expert on autogenic training Dr. Vladimir Levi comes to mind: "a mentally relaxed fist". (I wonder if Levi had heard the Zen koan: "Where does the fist disappear to when I open my hand?"). I strongly urge you to watch my DVD *Fast & Loose* to improve your relaxation skills.

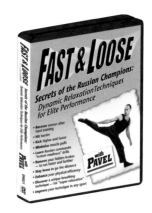

Eventually you will be capable of a rapid-fire, tight-loose-tight sequence—just like good punching. Just don't pick up the pace if you still have residual tension between reps! Alternate the hands and practice for a few hours a day, which is not as difficult as it sounds because you can carry the eraser with you anywhere you go.

The following passage from the "Karate Way" column in *Black Belt* by Dave Lowry will set you a distant goal to shoot for in this exercise, in your punches, and in your kettlebell swing:

> *Imagine a video of your reverse punch that's broken down into 10 frames. At what point do you begin to tighten the muscles you want to be firm so you make good, solid contact? A new student starts tightening as soon as the movement begins. He's self-conscious about the motion. He's trying to remember technical details. He's using all sorts of energy by squeezing his muscles long before his fist reaches the target. A more advanced practitioner, in contrast, stays loose and relaxed until frame No. 7 or No. 8. At higher levels, the tensing takes place at frame No. 10, the last moment. From there, more mastery comes when you don't tense at the beginning of No. 10 but at the last part of it.*

The karateka calls this ability "turning laziness into technical mastery". Note that this kind of "laziness" does not refer to slowing down or weakening the contraction but to limiting its duration, a very important Hardstyle distinction.

Some martial arts styles practice a very powerful Yang breathing technique called "reverse breathing". It calls for expanding the abdomen, especially the sides, when explosively exhaling and striking. Teaching it is beyond the scope of this book but various Zercher exercises will help you develop it.

Another excellent exercise to develop *kime* is the bottom-up kettlebell clean. Once you are proficient in the basic swing, place a light kettlebell slightly in front of you, its handle turned ninety degrees from what you are used to. Grip it exactly in the middle, hike it back, then swing it up to your chin level using your hips. Catch it bottom up by gripping the handle violently and tensing your abs. Drop the kettlebell back between your legs. Make sure to relax your arm. Several low rep sets totaling about 10 reps is all you need. This exercise does not tolerate fatigue. Eventually you may add bottom-up presses, front squats, and, if you are a stud like Max Shank, Senior RKC, even pistols to your arsenal. In addition to training *kime* and Yang breathing, bottom-up kettlebell drills forge a vise-like grip and unbendable wrists. Gray Cook also does some reflexive stabilization magic with them. For example, he improved the pullups of his wife Danielle Cook, RKCII who had problems firing one side of her abdominal wall, from 4 to 10 in one training session!

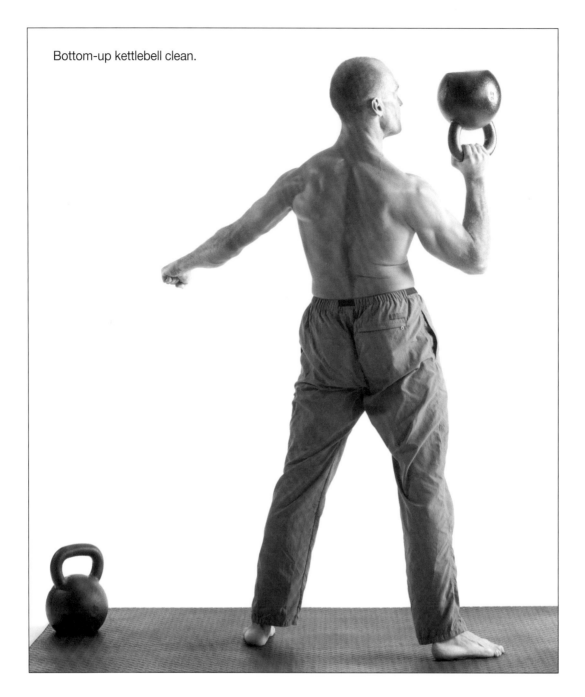

Bottom-up kettlebell clean.

Bottom-up cleans makes them a Yang exercise. The bottom-up kettlebell carry by Prof. McGill is pure Yin. He developed this drill after studying strongmen performing farmer's carries. The scientist realized how important were the quadratus lumborum, deep small muscles running up and down on both sides of the spine, to health and performance. The QL tilts the pelvis sideways and it essential not only to strongman but to the contact sport athletes. "Consider the footballer who plants the foot on a quick cut. A strong and stiff core assists the hip power to be transmitted up the body linkage with no energy losses resulting in a faster cut." For a fighter whose pelvis has to do all sorts of things during kicks the benefits are apparent. McGill prefers the bottom-up carry to the farmer's and racked versions because the BU enforces core stiffness—you will not be able to grip the bell without bracing. The professor promises that the drill will improve your "athleticism".

One of McGill's revolutionary midsection exercises for fighters combines Yin and Yang breathing: the latter is periodically overlaid on the former. Start spinning a ball on the end of a rope over your head. (Fill your wife's purse with something if you must, but don't use a kettlebell). The professor instructs: "As the ball passes 12 o'clock the athlete pulse-stiffens the body. Then switching to other times such as 3 o'clock trains neurological dexterity. The emphasis is on rapid contraction and relaxation."

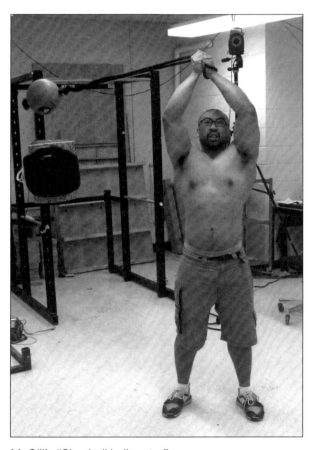 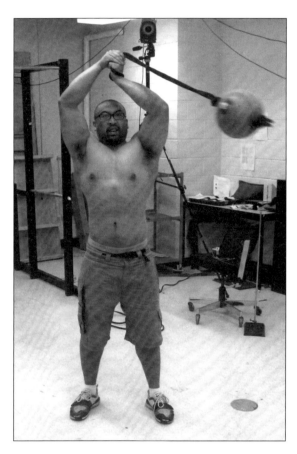

McGill's "Slamball helicopter".
Courtesy Prof. Stuart McGill's Spine Biomechanics Lab at the University of Waterloo, Canada

The above exercise is supposed to be done fast; sit-ups are not! Fast sit-ups not only ruin backs; they even have been known to injure the spinal cord and cause strokes! Don't go there.

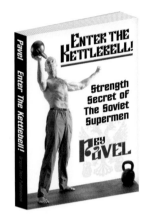

Enter the Kettlebell!
www.dragondoor.com/b33

One more suggestion for practicing both types of martial breathing while getting a whole lot of other benefits: Hardstyle kettlebell practice. Take our most fundamental routine: the Program Minimum from *Enter the Kettlebell!* It consists of only two exercises: the get-up and the swing. Doing the former for several minutes non-stop (switch hands after each rep though), especially with a heavy kettlebell is an excellent practice of Yin breathing. The other drill, the swing, is a Yang breathing practice, each rep performed with *kime*.

Among the many benefits of such training is a very special type of endurance. Recent research[65] has revealed a lot about the Hardstyle kettlebell "What the Hell Effect" when it concerns "conditioning." The author reviewed the existing research on respiratory muscles' fatigue and did his own. He found out that when these muscles get tired, they have a secondary unexpected and unpleasant effect on your ability to keep going. Metabolites in the diaphragm & Co. flick a switch in your nervous system that activates the fight-or-flight response and constricts blood vessels throughout the body. Therefore, "Respiratory muscle fatigue reduces limb blood flow, accelerates limb fatigue and increases limb effort perception." The good news is, according to the scientist, conditioning your breathing will increase your performance in many endurance activities.

Hardstyle Kettlebell Conditioning for Contact Sports

"Swings rock. Heavy swings rock more."

It is hard to disagree with David "the Iron Tamer" Whitley, Master RKC. According to Alison McConnell, the British scientist who authored the above "Respiratory Muscle Training as an Ergogenic Aid" study, conditioning your breathing muscles will increase your performance in many endurance activities without an increase in the VO2max and/or the lactate threshold. This might at least in part explain the WTHE of simple heavy kettlebell swing routines not optimized to raise these two parameters on endurance in contact sports.

Max Shank, Senior RKC, a fighter and all-around stud, makes heavy swings the foundation of his conditioning. His standard workout is 5min of one-arm swings with the

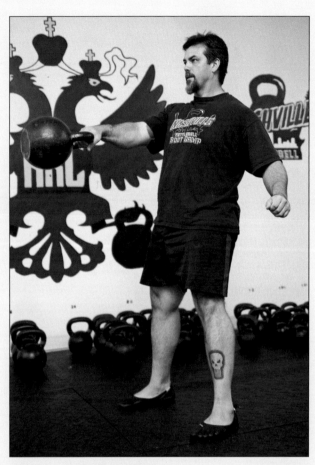

Photo courtesy David Whitley.

Beast, hitting 10 reps every time the clock beeps 30sec. This works out to about 100 swings total, 20 reps per minute and approximately 1:1 work to rest ratio. "If you throw in some finisher like this once or twice a week, you will be amazed at how everything you do starts to feel lighter and easier," promises Max.

"Swings are where it's at," writes Michael Castrogiovanni, RKC Team Leader, who has been with us almost since the very beginning of our RKC program and who is responsible for introducing the Russian kettlebell to NSCA. "They always have been and always will be! It is the foundation of kettlebell movements and anyone who invests significant amounts of time in themselves with the swing will reap great benefits and not only unlocks the secrets of their hips but the kettlebell as well. I agree with Max completely, it is what I have been saying for years and in fact it is how I prefer to train with kettlebells.

For one year I did nothing but swings, every which way, even though I had learned to clean and snatch, instinctively I knew the value in this foundational movement. After several months of swings I decided to return to wrestling, it had been a while due to injury (not from kettlebells) and I wanted to test the functionality and carryover of my newly forged strength. The two most important gains I noticed that translated from my training to the mat were: I was able to defend takedowns against guys who used to take me down at will, because I had more power and endurance in my sprawl. I also had longer lasting power endurance for takedowns late in the match when historically I would be too gassed to even attempt a takedown. I remember thinking how easy it was to maintain wrist control and how strange it was that my hands, wrists and forearms did not get sore despite my long break from wrestling."

Castro offers a few simple and powerful kettlebell swing routines.

The 10x10
Do 10 sets of 10 reps with a bell with as little rest as possible. If it is too easy, try another set; still too, easy add weight; still too easy add a bell. Try this protocol for 10 weeks. Stick with the same weight for 10 weeks and see what happens. 3 times a week

The 10x10 pyramid
Same as before, except increase your weight each set to five. Descend in weight for the last five.

The 10x10+10x10 diamond
Same as the pyramid but now go through the increase and decrease one more time to complete the Diamond.

Make sure you are outside and you have a place to throw the bell. After your 100th rep throw the bell as far as you can. This promotes that explosive endurance for the late in the game take down, when you don't think you've got anything left in the tank. Try it, practice it, you will be amazed!

"I have done almost every swing/snatch combo workout imaginable," states San Jose University head strength coach Chris Holder, RKC Team Leader, "and I always end up back to heavy swings…"

"Coach, I just don't get tired!" This is music to Chris' ears.

VO2max is not the only determinant of endurance.[66] For example, in the earlier mentioned studies of bicyclists and distance runners improving their endurance with heavy strength training, no change in maximal oxygen uptake was observed either. A serious athlete from a contact sport should address all aspects of his conditioning with appropriate methods: VO2max, lactate threshold, respiratory muscles' strength and endurance, absolute strength.

5. Provide reflexive rotary stability.

Item #5 on our list, rotary stability, refers to reflexive coordination of multi-plane movements engaging both the upper and the lower body. As Gray says, "You can't Hardstyle rotary stability". You may be strong as a bear in the full contact twist, yet if your core does not properly function reflexively, you will not be able to coordinate techniques like the Thai roundhouse kick well. Although rotary stability is developed by the kettlebell get-up, it may not be enough. Testing and correcting rotary stability is outside the scope of this book, refer to a CK-FMS instructor, www.dragondoor.com/instructors/ckfms_instructors/.

For Wrestlers and Grapplers

For obvious reasons grapplers need to be strong in the curled up in a ball position. A simple way to develop such strength while improving your pulling strength and making your

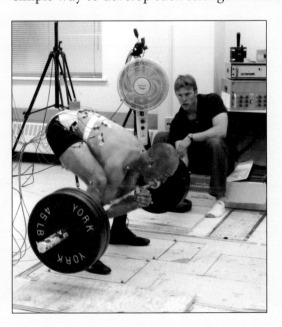

elbows healthier is to take a page from the book of Steve Baccari, RKC and do chin-ups finished by curling up in a ball and holding this position.

Wrestlers need be able to lift their opponents from very uncomfortable positions. The Zercher deadlift (see the photo) is a dangerous yet effective exercise. Alexander Karelin has done 440x10! Although the upper back will unavoidably flex, do your best to keep your lower back flat and "hinge" through your hips.

Courtesy Prof. Stuart McGill's Spine Biomechanics Lab at the University of Waterloo, Canada

If all of the above seems overwhelming and complicated, just follow the *Enter the Kettlebell!* Program Minimum with a heavy kettlebell, eventually 32-48kg. Yes, it is that simple.

FOOTNOTES

58 Støren et al. (2008). Thanks to Chad Waterbury for pointing this study out to me.

59 Sunde et al. (2010)

60 deVries (1980)

61 McCloskey et al. (1983)

62 Cafarelli (1982)

63 McConnell (2009). I would like to thank Jeremy Layport for bringing this paper to my attention.

64 Dickerman et al. (2005)

65 McConnell (2009)

66 McConnell (2009)

ABOUT PAVEL

Pavel Tsatsouline, is a former Soviet Special Forces physical training instructor, currently a subject matter expert to the US Navy SEALs and the US Secret Service.

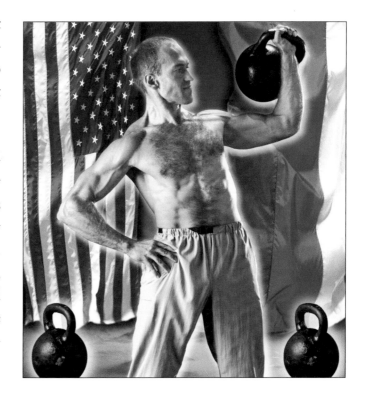

Although Pavel's expertise lies in training gun carrying professionals, his "low tech/high concept" training methods have been increasingly and successfully used by elite athletes and their coaches. Among them are UFC star Joe Lauzon, 200m sprint women's world record holder Allyson Felix, and Donnie Thompson who posted the highest powerlifting total of all time.

Pavel is the author of several bestselling strength training books, including *Power to the People!, The Naked Warrior,* and *Enter the Kettlebell!*

In 2001 Pavel's company and Dragon Door introduced the Russian kettlebell to the West and launched RKC, the kettlebell instructor course, which became the industry's golden standard.

Abs for Shock and Awe

How to Develop the Ultimate in Wrought-Iron Muscle, Mid-Section Body Armor and Core Generation of Explosive Power

The sole goal of *Hardstyle Abs* is to achieve an extraordinarily strong mid-section. But not simply to swivel heads with your rippling "six-pack". For, according to Pavel, your abs should be simultaneously weapon, armor and force generator. The six-pack is just a side effect of the coiled power with which you now operate.

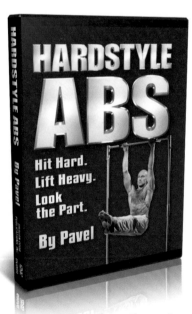

2 Mid-Level

3 Advanced

Hardstyle Abs
Hit Hard. Lift Heavy. Look the Part.
By Pavel
#DV089   **$29.95**
DVD Running time: 29 minutes

Hardstyle Abs will give you impenetrable body armor—to withstand a direct hit of the greatest magnitude. *Hardstyle Abs* will give you the generative force to retaliate with a devastating backlash. And *Hardstyle Abs* will help you lift more weight than ever before—more safely.

After years of dedicated research and experimentation, Pavel has identified three "killer" drills, as all you need to achieve this level of mid-section mastery. Follow Pavel's battle plan to the T and the results are guaranteed—noticeable within weeks, extraordinary within months. Pavel provides the laser focus. You? Simply obey the commands.

Discover:

- Why high reps have failed you—and the "secret sauce" that will have your abs tuned for heavy action all day long and at a moment's notice.

- Hardstyle breathing—for explosive power and a bullet-proof waist.

- The Hardstyle Sit-up—to generate an unbelievable contraction for superior results.

- Internal Isometrics—the lost secret behind the old-time physical culturalists' exceptional abdominal strength and development.

- The Hardstyle Hanging Leg Raise—the final weapon you must master to channel the power of your every muscle into one devastating surge.

Just <u>five reps a day</u> is all it takes...

"Unique Ab Pavelizer II™ smokes your abs more intensely, safely and quickly than any abs machine in the world—guaranteed!"

The Ab Pavelizer II™'s sleek design guarantees a perfect sit-up by forcing you to do it right. Now, escape or half-measures are impossible. Sit down at the Ab Pavelizer II™ and a divine slab of abs will be served up whether you like it or not. You'll startle yourself in your own mirror!

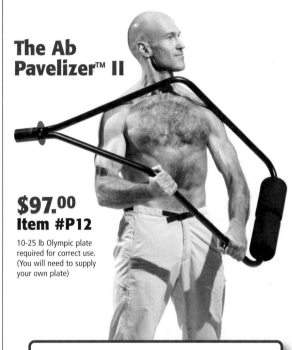

The Ab Pavelizer™ II

$97.00
Item #P12

10-25 lb Olympic plate required for correct use. (You will need to supply your own plate)

"I work my abs a lot and they are probably stronger than the average guy but I found out just how pathetic they were when my Pavelizer arrived. This is an amazingly effective piece of equipment. By taking the hip flexors out of play and isolating the abs, they have to work like never before. Combined with the power breathing, my abs are getting stronger by the day."—**Charles Long**, Burlington, CO

"The Ab Pavelizer is hands down "THE" best AB training device I have ever used! Simple put, this thing is evil! I noticed almost immediate results and a burn in my AB's that I never thought possible! I have better six pack AB's at 28yrs. old than I did when I was 19! If you want to melt your mid-section and destroy those love handles, the Ab Pavelizer is the one tool that gets it done in a hurry!"—**Sean, Lacey**, WA

"The Ab Pavelizer really is the best thing to do for your abs. I've been doing kettlebells for a while and am in pretty good shape, but this is really starting to make my abs visible.

This product isn't cheap, but when you consider it (a) gives you stronger, more visible abs guaranteed (b) improves your overall kettlebell strength/proficiency (c) gives you better posture and probably saves you money in chiropractor visits and (d) lasts forever. Considering all this its well worth the price."
—**Tony, Santa Monica**, CA

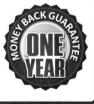

How sure are we that Ab Pavelizer™ II will work for you? If you are not 100% absolutely thrilled with your purchase, Dragon Door Publications will refund of your entire purchase price for up to a FULL YEAR!

MONEY BACK GUARANTEE
ONE YEAR

FREE BONUS:

Comes with a four page detailed instruction guide on how to use and get the most out of your Ab Pavelizer™ II. Includes two incredible methods for massively intensifying your ab workout with Power and Paradox Breathing.

www.dragondoor.com
1•800•899•5111

Dragon Door

Order *Ab Pavelizer* online:
www.dragondoor.com/P12

Are Rigid Muscles Robbing You of Your Strength?

Traditional stretching programs weaken you — but stop stretching altogether and you'll doom yourself to injuries and mediocrity. Discover the world's only stretching protocol specifically and uniquely designed to increase—not reduce—a powerlifter's strength. Skyrocket your strength now—and reduce the wear and tear on your joints—by mastering the secrets of *Strength Stretching!*

- **How to gain** up to 15% on your pulling strength
- **How to arch higher**—and bench more—without killing your back
- **Master the Kettlebell Depth Squat** — the Russian powerlifting secret for teaching perfect squat and pull form and developing championship flexibility
- **Discover how** to release the hidden brakes that are silently sabotaging your deadlift
- **How to relax** your turtle traps—and up your dead
- **How to squat with the big boys**—without killing your shoulders and elbows

Strength Stretching
For a Bigger Squat, Bench & Deadlift
with Pavel
#DV024 $39.95
DVD Running time: 38 minutes

2 Mid-Level
3 Advanced

"Strength Stretching is a virtual must for the powerlifter, novice or advanced. Strength Stretching has helped **Westside Barbell** enormously and I know it will help everyone who is in powerlifting at any stage of the game."
—*Louie Simmons,* Westside Barbell

"**Pavel** is a fitness visionary. He has been teaching people about whole body functional training when sports scientists and exercise leaders were emphasizing aerobics and muscle isolation bodybuilding techniques. He formulated his methods by combining training principles developed by Soviet and eastern European coaches and scientists, worldwide sports medicine research, and personal experience. His books and DVDs will help athletes increase power, functional flexibility, and neuromuscular control, while minimizing the risk of injury. Coaches, athletes, and sports scientists will benefit from his unique training courses."
—*DR. THOMAS FAHEY, Exercise Physiology Lab, Dept of Kinesiology Track and Field Team, California State University, Chico*

Discover your body's true potential
"Pavel instructs on many crucial points in an exemplary precise and detailed way, making them very easy to grasp, follow and most importantly gain from. Having been in the game for quite a while, I thought I had reached a plateau near my max potential, but within a month of applying his advice I have added 33% to all the three majors - bench, squat and dead and I'm confident the gains will continue: *Strength Stretching* is a roadmap to the adventure of rediscovering the body and its true potential. I strongly recommend it to any powerlifter, serious fitness athlete or personal trainer."
—**Kim Bach Petersen**, Denmark

I just thought I knew how to squat!
"I've been squatting for 18 years and have spent the last 8 years teaching young football players the squat. I realized only a few minutes into the DVD that I really didn't know as much about squatting as I thought I did. I had bought the DVD to help with my hip flexibility and got so much more than just that. It was worth the price and will continue to pay dividends in the future. If you're serious about any or all of the three power lifts this DVD is a must have resource!"
—**Darren Lamar**, High School Football Coach, Temple, OK

"Pavel's stretching ability is unbelievable. As World Class as it comes!"
—*Brad Gillingham,* 2 times World Superheavyweight Powerlifting Champion

"I loved the DVD. A viewer might discover that they may already be doing several of the Strength Stretches but might quickly discover, as I did, that one additional idea or factor can turn that stretch into a game changer. Good Stuff!"
—*Dan John,* **National Masters Champion in Discus and Olympic Lifting, Salt Lake City, UT**

"When I consume a teaching resource, I look for two things; first does it have something I can use immediately, and second does it mention something that I have been playing with in the gym. *Strength Stretching* hits both points several times. Great for both new and more experienced PLers. Very few things have my full endorsement, but this does."
—*Jack Reape,* **Armed Forces Powerlifting Champion**

Be as FLEXIBLE as You Want to Be—FASTER, SAFER and SOONER

Relax Into Stretch is for people who want to be [bo]th flexible and strong, and the principles it will [te]ach you can help you stay strong and injury-free in [all] the activities of your daily life, not just stretching. [I h]ad a severely herniated lumbar disc a few years [bac]k; Pavel's *Power To The People!* was the [be]ginning of my salvation, *Russian Kettlebell [C]hallenge* taught me to add endurance and some [fle]xibility to my strength, and Relax Into Stretch was [the] icing on the cake, teaching me how to go from [no]t being able to touch my toes to being able to do [sp]lits within the space of 6 months while almost 50 [ye]ars old!"—Steve Freides, Ridgewood, NJ

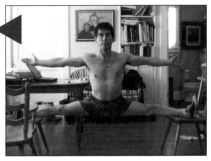

Picture of me in a split - that says it all, and I owe it all to *Relax Into Stretch*. –Steve

The Stretching Bible

"This book tells you HOW and WHY and WHEN to stretch. The photos make it easy to learn the various stretches. This book allows anyone to customize their own stretching program to exactly what their own focus needs to be. I use it as a powerlifter, my wife uses it as a dancer, my boss even used it to get ready to take a ski vacation. A must for every athlete."
—Jack Reape, New Orleans, LA

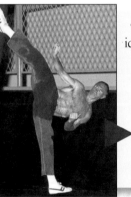

"Pavel has great ideas on flexibility and strength exercises."
—Bill "Superfoot" Wallace, M.Sc., World Kickboxing Champion

Stop wasting your stretching time!

"Pavel lines out more information on stretching than I got during the entire 6 years I spent earning a Bachelor's degree in exercise physiology and Master's in physical therapy! The information is clear, easy to read, and works like a charm! I've stretched fairly aggressively over the years with the knowledge I had, but I've made significant gains over the past couple weeks with the information contained on these pages! If you want to do the splits you should get this book!"—Jason Goumas, Lexington, KY

Terrific program—explains all you need!

"A great program for martial arts stretching and stretching for health and wellness! No more back or joint pain. Full leg splits in all four directions within just a few weeks."—Joshua Hatcher, Newington CT, USA

Best stretching book

"When I first read this book, I was 6 inches from doing a full side split and couldn't go down any further. After six weeks of using the principles contained in this book in my own flexibility training, I did my first full side split."—Mercer, NL, Canada

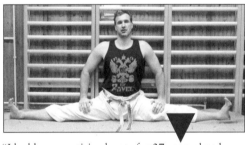

"I had been practicing karate for 27 years already when I learned about Pavel Tsatsouline's stretching books. By that time I totally gave up on a side split. But in these books I read about completely different things, than that I was used to… It took 3 months to achieve my goal …at the age of 41."
—Dr. Zolnai Vilmos, RKC II, Hungarian Shotokan Karate

- Own an illustrated guide to the thirty-six most effective techniques for super-flexibility
- How the secret of mastering your emotions can add immediate inches to your stretch
- How to wait out your tension—the surprising key to greater mobility and a better stretch
- How to fool your reflexes into giving you all the stretch you want
- Why *contract-relax stretching* is 267% more effective than conventional relaxed stretching
- How to breathe your way to greater flexibility

- Using the Russian technique of *Forced Relaxation* as your ultimate stretching weapon
- How to stretch when injured—faster, safer ways to heal
- Young, old, male, female—learn what stretches are best for you and what stretches to avoid
- Why excessive flexibility can be detrimental to athletic performance—and how to determine your real flexibility needs
- Plateau-busting strategies for the chronically inflexible.

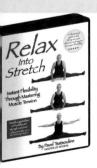
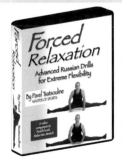
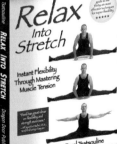
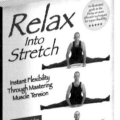

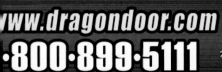
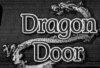

Acclaim for *The Naked Warrior*

"If I was stuck on a desert island (or somewhere else with no access to weights) I'd hope that Pavel Tsatsouline would be there to help keep me in shape. With *The Naked Warrior*, Pavel has moved the art of exercise without weights to a new level. I like both the exercises he has selected and the approach he advocates for training on them. Now, whether you have weights or not, there is no reason not to get into top shape!"
—Arthur Drechsler, author *The Weightlifting Encyclopedia*

"*The Naked Warrior* is one of Pavel's best works yet!!! I find that Pavel's easy to understand, no nonsense approach will help one become the best they can be. In addition, the tools Pavel explains will help my Olympic style weight lifters gain the core strength they need to put additional kg on their totals. Thanks, Pavel, for such a great work!!"
—Mike Burgener, Senior international weightlifting coach

Enter Warriors Only Circle

"For those of you who read, my hat goes off to you. For those of you who actually apply what you read are priceless actions from noble spirits. *The Naked Warrior* is a book for True Warriors, not you people who thought that they could get results by just reading. This book is by far second to none. *The Naked Warrior* focuses on meat and potatoes to increase your strength, not getting big. For the record, true warriors need to be as strong, slim and trim as you can, yet not huge. We have to be full of fight, violence of action, all

the time, every time. (Low weight is a HUGE factor in the Special Operations World / Airborne. Hence, we can hold so much gear factored into the lift capabilities of the aircraft we are deployed in.) Think about it: would you like to have the same power as a guy who is 3 times your size? I challenge you to apply what you read and follow the training faithfully. We don't have time to train wrong."
—Sal "Ghost Wolf 6" Sagev, Ft. Bragg, NC

Delivers better results than I could have hoped for!

"*The Naked Warrior* is an outstanding book. Using its principles not only delivers results, but delivers them super quickly. I used the techniques to get from 8 to 18 chinups using the "Grease the Groove" method described in the book in 3 WEEKS! My previous lifetime best being 12 chinups. I am also gaining substantial increase in muscle mass in my chest, arms and back."
—Mike Harrop, London, England

Pavel has done a fantastic job on this book, a must read for all

"I briefly want to say that I will be forever grateful to Pavel and his real world knowledge of the body and what it takes to really get in shape. I'm a 53 year old two tour former Marine Sgt. Listen, I had knee surgery a little over a year ago and have tried everything to get my strength back and nothing has worked—until now! Pavel, man you have blown me away with this program. Not just my

knees but my whole body are stronger by the week… Pavel can put you back in the game!"
—Gene Simmons, New Jersey

Continuous progress with GTG

"Before I started the "Grease the Groove" program, my personal record in pullups was 18. I am glad to say after only three weeks of GTG, I knocked off 25 pullups. I am trying to go through in my head what just happened, because while on this program I would never be sore and never even break a sweat. I just complete my fourth week as of yesterday and tested my max again… 28 pullups. If I would have discovered this years ago, I could very well be in the 40's, even 50's, in pullups!"
—Jason W. Masangkay, Orlando, FL

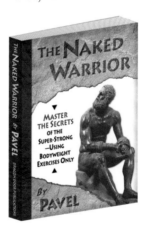

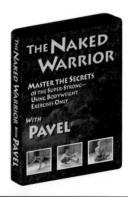

You just thought you knew about bodyweight exercises!

"Pavel's DVD is a treasure trove of information for any beginner or expert strength trainer. I was trained by Bill Starr in powerlifting and weightlifting and was a personal trainer/instructor 26 years, Military Police/ Correctional Officer for 11 years and coaching/instructing Judo and Ju-jitsu for the last 8 years, and I was in the Marine Corps, Navy, and the Guard for giggles and grins, so I have some knowledge on the subject matter. I can honestly say that Pavel is 100% correct! Give his DVD or book a shot (hell, I bought both!) and you'll see that you don't need hundreds of reps or dozens of different exercises to become rock hard and strong as coiled steel."
—James Copelin, Texoma Judo-Jujitsu, Wichita Falls, TX

The Naked Warrior
Master the Secrets of the Super-Strong —Using Bodyweight Exercises Only
By Pavel
#B28 $39.95
Paperback   218 pages   8.5" x 11"
Over 190 black & white photos plus several illustrations

The Naked Warrior
Master the Secrets of the Super-Strong —Using Bodyweight Exercises Only
with Pavel
DVD   **#DV015 $34.95**
Running time 37 minutes

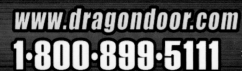

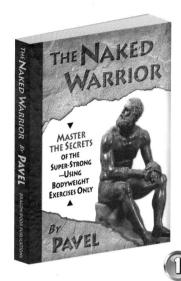
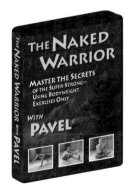

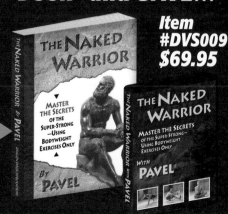

Discover New Keys to Superior Athletic Achievement

In his strength books Pavel emphasizes the importance of learning to maximally tense the muscles. Because tension IS strength. But strength/ tension is only half of the total performance package. The other half is relaxation. The body of a karate expert will freeze in total tension at the moment of impact, but will remain totally loose before and after.

Mastery of relaxation is the hallmark of an elite athlete. Soviet scientists discovered that the higher the athlete's level, the quicker he can relax his muscles. The Soviets observed an 800% difference between novices and Olympians. Their conclusion: total control of tension = elite performance.

If you can master your muscular tension, a new dimension of athletic excellence opens to you. New achievements. New heights of performance. Some genetically-endowed superstars seem to possess this ability from birth. But according to former Soviet Special Forces trainer, Pavel, a SKILL–SET is available that can transform *anyone's* current physical limitations.

Now, for the first time, Pavel reveals these little known Soviet performance secrets, so you too can become the master of your body — not its victim. From years of research and experience, Pavel has selected these *Fast & Loose* techniques as the best-of-the-best for practical and quick results.

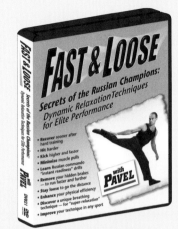

Mandatory for the serious fighter "I've spent the last couple of years desperately trying to recover the speed I've been losing by inches. Before I'd even finished watching this DVD, it became clear what I'd really lost. Years ago, I used to 'snap' strikes in. As I've become a more serious fighter, I've succumbed to trying to 'drive' them in (karateka can read this as misunderstanding what it really means to train "with kime"). It's ironic that the fact that I'm trying so much harder is what has been slowing me down all along. I credit Pavel for explaining this so clearly & demonstrating drills that deliver rapid results. If you're a serious competitor looking for that extra edge, you *must* add these drills to your routine. Thank you, Pavel, for another excellent product. OSU!!" —B, Boston, MA

Fast & Loose
Secrets of the Russian Champions: Dynamic Relaxation Techniques for Elite Performance
with Pavel
#DV021 $29.95
DVD Running time:
27 minutes

Mid-Level

Advanced

Fast and Loose + Rough and Tough = Deadly Force

Invest in the "Deadly Force" set of Pavel's *Fast and Loose* DVD with Pavel's *The Naked Warrior* DVD and book— and SAVE...

Item #DVS008
$94.85

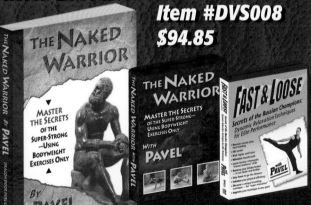

- Recover sooner after hard training
- Kick higher and faster
- Hit harder
- Minimize muscle pulls
- Stay loose to go the distance
- Improve your technique in any sport

- Enhance your physical efficiency
- Remove your hidden brakes — to run faster and further
- Learn Russian commando "instant readiness" drills
- Discover a unique breathing technique — for "super-relaxation"

"Fast & Loose is another amazing tool from Pavel... Everyone knows that once you really start pushing the envelope on your current abilities, you need those subtle yet all-important tools to move from average to elite performance. They can seem insignificant to the untrained observer, but are better than gold to those who have the faculties to incorporate them. Pavel delivers as always."
—Mark Hanington, Huntington Beach, CA.

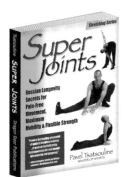
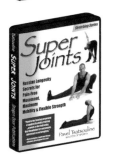

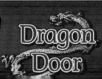

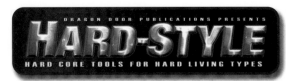

DRAGON DOOR PUBLICATIONS PRESENTS

HARD CORE TOOLS FOR HARD LIVING TYPES

1·800·899·5111
24 HOURS A DAY
FAX YOUR ORDER (866) 280-7619

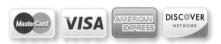
MasterCard VISA AMERICAN EXPRESS DISCOVER NETWORK

O R D E R I N G   I N F O R M A T I O N

Customer Service Questions? Please call us between 9:00am– 11:00pm EST Monday to Friday at 1-800-899-5111. Local and foreign customers call 214-258-0134 for orders and customer service

100% One-Year Risk-Free Guarantee. If you are not completely satisfied with any product—we'll be happy to give you a prompt exchange, credit, or refund, as you wish. Simply return your purchase to us,

and please let us know why you were dissatisfied—it will help us to provide better products and services in the future. *Shipping and handling fees are non-refundable.*

Telephone Orders For faster service you may place your orders by calling Toll Free 24 hours a day, 7 days a week, 365 days per year. When you call, please have your credit card ready.

Complete and mail with full payment to: Dragon Door Publications, 5 County Road B East, Suite 3, Little Canada, MN 55117

Please print clearly

Sold To: **A**

Name_____

Street _____

City _____

State _____ Zip _____

Day phone*_____
* Important for clarifying questions on orders

Please print clearly

SHIP TO: *(Street address for delivery)*   **B**

Name_____

Street _____

City _____

State _____ Zip _____

Email _____

ITEM #	QTY.	ITEM DESCRIPTION	ITEM PRICE	A OR B	TOTAL

HANDLING AND SHIPPING CHARGES— FOR MAIL ORDERS ONLY

Phone orders—your Dragon Door representative will give you the exact price
Website orders—shipping and handling will display automatically

Total Amount of Order Add (Excludes kettlebells and kettlebell kits):

$00.00 to 29.99	Add $7.30	$100.00 to 129.99	Add $15.70
$30.00 to 49.99	Add $8.35	$130.00 to 169.99	Add $17.80
$50.00 to 69.99	Add $9.40	$170.00 to 199.99	Add $19.90
$70.00 to 99.99	Add $12.55	$200.00 to 299.99	Add $22.00
		$300.00 and up	Add $26.20

Canada and Mexico double the charges; All other countries triple the charges.

Total of Goods	
Shipping Charges	
Rush Charges	
Kettlebell Shipping Charges	
TX residents add 8.25% sales tax	
MN residents add 7.125% sales tax	
TOTAL ENCLOSED	

METHOD OF PAYMENT ❏ CHECK ❏ M.O. ❏ MASTERCARD ❏ VISA ❏ DISCOVER ❏ AMEX

Account No. *(Please indicate all numbers on your credit card)*   EXPIRATION DATE   CCV

☐☐☐☐ ☐☐☐☐ ☐☐☐☐ ☐☐☐☐   ☐☐/☐☐   ☐☐☐

Day Phone: (   ) _____

Signature: _____ **Date:** _____

NOTE: *We ship best method available for your delivery address. Foreign orders are sent by air. Credit card or International M.O. only. For* **RUSH** *processing of your order, add an additional $10.00 per address. Available on money order & charge card orders only.*

Errors and omissions excepted. Prices subject to change without notice.

Warning to foreign customers: **The Customs in your country may or may not tax or otherwise charge you an additional fee for goods you receive. Dragon Door Publications is charging you only for U.S. handling and international shipping. Dragon Door Publications is in no way responsible for any additional fees levied by Customs, the carrier or any other entity.**

Warning!
This may be the last issue of the catalog you receive.

If we rented your name, or you haven't ordered in the last two years you may not hear from us again. If you wish to stay informed about products and services that can make a difference to your health and well-being, please indicate below.

Name _____

Address _____

City _____ State _____ Zip _____

Phone _____

Do You Have A Friend Who'd Like To Receive This Catalog?

We would be happy to send your friend a free copy. Make sure to print and complete in full:

Name _____

Address _____

City _____ State _____ Zip _____

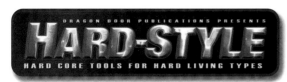

ORDERING INFORMATION

Customer Service Questions? Please call us between 9:00am– 11:00pm EST Monday to Friday at 1-800-899-5111. Local and foreign customers call 214-258-0134 for orders and customer service

100% One-Year Risk-Free Guarantee. If you are not completely satisfied with any product—we'll be happy to give you a prompt exchange, credit, or refund, as you wish. Simply return your purchase to us,

and please let us know why you were dissatisfied—it will help us to provide better products and services in the future. *Shipping and handling fees are non-refundable.*

Telephone Orders For faster service you may place your orders by calling Toll Free 24 hours a day, 7 days a week, 365 days per year. When you call, please have your credit card ready.

1·800·899·5111
24 HOURS A DAY
FAX YOUR ORDER (866) 280-7619

Complete and mail with full payment to: Dragon Door Publications, 5 County Road B East, Suite 3, Little Canada, MN 55117

Please print clearly

Sold To: **A**

Name_____

Street_____

City_____

State _____ Zip _____

Day phone*_____
* Important for clarifying questions on orders

Please print clearly

SHIP TO: *(Street address for delivery)*   **B**

Name_____

Street_____

City_____

State _____ Zip _____

Email_____

ITEM #	QTY.	ITEM DESCRIPTION	ITEM PRICE	A OR B	TOTAL

HANDLING AND SHIPPING CHARGES— FOR MAIL ORDERS ONLY

Phone orders–your Dragon Door representative will give you the exact price
Website orders–shipping and handling will display automatically

Total Amount of Order Add (Excludes kettlebells and kettlebell kits):

$00.00 to 29.99	Add $7.30	$100.00 to 129.99	Add $15.70
$30.00 to 49.99	Add $8.35	$130.00 to 169.99	Add $17.80
$50.00 to 69.99	Add $9.40	$170.00 to 199.99	Add $19.90
$70.00 to 99.99	Add $12.55	$200.00 to 299.99	Add $22.00
		$300.00 and up	Add $26.20

Canada and Mexico double the charges; All other countries triple the charges.

Total of Goods	
Shipping Charges	
Rush Charges	
Kettlebell Shipping Charges	
TX residents add 8.25% sales tax	
MN residents add 7.125% sales tax	
TOTAL ENCLOSED	

METHOD OF PAYMENT ❏ CHECK ❏ M.O. ❏ MASTERCARD ❏ VISA ❏ DISCOVER ❏ AMEX

Account No. *(Please indicate all numbers on your credit card)*   EXPIRATION DATE   CCV

☐☐☐☐ ☐☐☐☐ ☐☐☐☐ ☐☐☐☐   ☐☐/☐☐   ☐☐☐

Day Phone: (   ) _____

Signature: _____ **Date:** _____

NOTE: *We ship best method available for your delivery address. Foreign orders are sent by air. Credit card or International M.O. only. For* **RUSH** *processing of your order, add an additional $10.00 per address. Available on money order & charge card orders only.*

Errors and omissions excepted. Prices subject to change without notice.

Warning to foreign customers:
The Customs in your country may or may not tax or otherwise charge you an additional fee for goods you receive. Dragon Door Publications is charging you only for U.S. handling and international shipping. Dragon Door Publications is in no way responsible for any additional fees levied by Customs, the carrier or any other entity.

Warning!
This may be the last issue of the catalog you receive.

If we rented your name, or you haven't ordered in the last two years you may not hear from us again. If you wish to stay informed about products and services that can make a difference to your health and well-being, please indicate below.

Name_____

Address_____

City _____ State _____ Zip _____

Phone_____

Do You Have A Friend Who'd Like To Receive This Catalog?

We would be happy to send your friend a free copy. Make sure to print and complete in full:

Name_____

Address_____

City _____ State _____ Zip _____